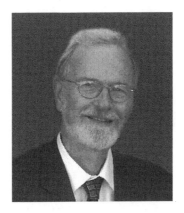

## About the Author

Mike Shirk studied Engineering and English Literature at Purdue University, Marketing at Wayne State University and Business Administration at National University. He spent most of his life working as an advertising copywriter and creative director. Thus he had the perfect background to prepare him for the challenges of dealing with an incurable, progressive, neuromuscular disease. This is his first book but he hopes it will not be his last.

*To Janet and Rich*
*from Mike*

i

# Rolling Back

## Through a Life Disabled

*By Mike Shirk*

*ISBN-13: 978-1495389825*

*ISBN-10: 1495389820*

*Copyright © 2014 Mike Shirk*

*Cover Image ©2009 Elizabeth Shirk*

*http://lifedisabled.com*

## Dedication

*This book is dedicated to my late wife, Beth Shirk and to my children who have been forced to roll along on this journey through disability. Instead of being supported by a strong father to help them build their own lives, they have been called upon to provide support far earlier than they could have possibly imagined.*

Mike Shirk

# Rolling Back

## Through a Life Disabled

# Contents

# To My Readers

Many years ago I would have loved to have found this book. I had been diagnosed with a rare form of muscle disease called inclusion body myositis and had no idea what to expect. If I could roll back time, my life would have turned out much differently. I would have done a much better job of preparing for what lay ahead. I could have avoided being blindsided by changes I didn't see coming. I would have traveled more and worried about money less, hugged my wife and children more, because I would have known there would come a day when I could not.

Going by the philosophy of better late than never, I have written *Rolling Back* to give myself advice should they perfect time travel in the next few years. Perhaps you or someone you know, or especially, someone you care for has been diagnosed with a disabling disease, suffered a stroke, or had a paralyzing injury. If so, this might be the book you need.

I was diagnosed with inclusion body myositis in 1996, although I suffered from its effects for many years before. Just when I was learning to adapt, my wife was diagnosed with her own rare and untreatable disease - myotonic muscular dystrophy. Our diseases were similar in the way they took away our ability to walk, to use our hands in a skillful manner (a serious issue since we were both artists) and they seemed to force us to rethink our living arrangements every other week. This book is about the things we learned and that I am still learning by myself now that my wife has passed away. I've shared some of this information with the tens of thousands of people who have visited my Life Disabled blog. You will find references to parts of that blog sprinkled here and there, as it is filled with pictures, illustrations and videos that couldn't be included here.

I hope you find *Rolling Back* to be interesting, sometimes entertaining, but always helpful.

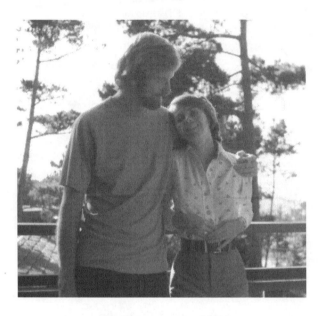

*On Honeymoon, 1974*

# Prologue

As our rental car rolled backward down the narrow mountain road, I thought to myself, "This won't end well." We had driven to the top of Mount Haleakala on Maui during a family vacation when the engine vapor locked and wouldn't start. The only cure was to get to lower altitude, but we were facing uphill. So we backed down a couple of miles with no power steering or brakes. That was an adventure, because we survived and didn't even have to buy the rental agency a new car. But the years with two untreatable progressive illnesses have been worse, because we knew what was waiting at the bottom of the hill.

From the moment we met until death separated us, my wife and I traveled a path carved by remarkable coincidences. Our first 25 years were a beautiful love story that I might tell someday, but not now. This is the story of our last 15 years, when two rare illnesses took us down a road with no signposts, no guardrails, and no return.

Being diagnosed with a rare disease like inclusion body myositis can be a bit frightening. I think a lot of that has to do with the feeling you are alone. At the time I didn't know if there would be anyone in all of San Diego who might share it. Later, I would learn that there were actually several of us. Even so, day-to-day life with a disease such as this can be lonely. Friends and family want to help, but they can't fully understand what you are going through. I hope this book may serve as a source of companionship for others who are living with a rare disease or disability. If you are caring for such a person, you may find information here that will give you new insight into their challenges.

I lived both roles after my wife was diagnosed with myotonic muscular dystrophy, but my experience as a caregiver was somewhat different since I was also dealing with my own illness.

You won't find medical advice here; I am not a medical professional. But, as many with rare diseases have discovered, you quickly become an expert in your "specialty" because there are so few people studying it in medical school or in practice. With that in mind, I have included some information gleaned from my personal research here and there. Part of it is based on peer-reviewed studies and articles that I have found in the medical literature. Some of it is my own best estimate of a situation. In either case, please see your doctor or confirm the facts for yourself. I've included resources in the back to help you.

Another goal of this book is to provide information about the tools and techniques needed to cope with a degenerative muscle disease. I will tell you about the adaptations I made over the course of my journey, beginning with a walking stick, and ending where I am today, in an assisted living facility with caregivers using an overhead hoist to move me. In between, there have been literally dozens of different adaptive devices that I have tried, some of which were very useful, some of which were not.

I like to tell stories now and then. I think they help make my points. So if you will bear with me, I have a story right now.

# Warning Signs

It was midmorning on a sunny day in San Diego. I had been running for more than three and a half hours and was now grinding my way up the dreaded five-mile climb along Friars Road. It was the same route that the Spanish Missionaries followed in 1774 when they moved their original Mission away from the coast and five miles inland along the San Diego River. But this was 1983, and I was nearing the entrance to the stadium where the San Diego Marathon would finish. I was so tired and in such pain that for a few seconds I stopped running and considered calling it quits. But then I thought about the months of training I had endured to reach this point. Getting up each morning well before sunrise, running from my home several miles to the west to Mission Bay, making a lap around Fiesta Island and returning home in time to shower and get ready for work. Most days I would run at least 10 miles, sometimes 20, to prepare for my first full marathon. Determined to finish what I had started, I began running again, each foot plant sending pain through the length of my body.

A few minutes later, I turned into the stadium parking lot and soon crossed the finish line, joining the throng of several thousand runners and well-wishers. Instead of celebrating my finish with the rest of the participants, I focused on getting away from the bustle. But I was so exhausted and confused that I could not even find my way out of the stadium to my car. A Red Cross worker noted my dazed expression and asked if I needed medical help. I told her I just needed to find the exit. With a perplexed look, she pointed to it – clearly marked, and further identified by a large column of departing runners and spectators.

Several weeks later, back at work, I was finding it very hard to do my job. The fever I had experienced for several days post-race was gone, but I still ached from head to toe and felt nauseous much of the time. I had always been able to shake off illness in the past, so it surprised me that this had hung on so long. To this day, I wonder if I inflicted some permanent damage on my immune system by running that marathon. Could it have led to my disability?

A few years later, I was shooting baskets at a client's home. Every shot I took fell about a foot short of the rim. I asked if it had been installed higher than regulation and he assured me that it had been accurately measured. "Curious," I thought. "Was my aim off that much?"

After the marathon, I resumed running, although shorter distances. I would usually run about five miles and try to average seven to eight minutes a mile. My times were getting worse and I wondered why. I began keeping track of my training schedule on an Excel spreadsheet. I accumulated a couple of years' data, and the results were clear - no matter how much I trained, my running speed was steadily declining.

Many times when I would return from a run, my pants would be torn and my legs would be bloody. Was I running in a tough neighborhood? No, I would stumble and fall somewhere along the route. The slightest bit of uneven pavement would cause me to trip. Unable to catch myself, I would fall. I chalked it up to being clumsy, not realizing it was a sign of weakening quadriceps muscles.

I was also a golfer. Sometime in the early 1990s, I

noticed my driving distance was decreasing, even after I switched to the most modern clubs and balls available. On the driving range I would often lose my grip on the club and it would sail 50 yards away. My hands were obviously getting weaker as well.

Each of these problems could be linked to either weak quadriceps muscles or weak finger flexors, classic signs of a rare muscle disease. My doctor showed little interest but said he would check for a thyroid problem. My thyroid tested fine and the doctor said my symptoms were normal aging. I was still in my early fifties!

I can't blame him entirely. Primary care doctors deal with a huge range of conditions and have limited training in specialized fields such as neuromuscular diseases. If I thought something was wrong, I should have insisted on a referral to a specialist.

# Getting Diagnosed

One day everything changed. I had taken a nap in an awkward position and twisted my neck. I thought it would get better by the next day, but instead it was worse and so painful to raise my head I barely managed the drive to urgent care. A doctor I had never seen before was on duty. She examined my neck and said I just had a spasm that could be relieved with an anti-inflammatory. It was a fairly short visit to that point, until I stood up to leave.

Without thinking, I placed my hands on the arms of the chair and pushed myself upright. She saw me out of the corner of her eye and asked me to stop.

"Why did you get up that way?" she asked.

"What way?"

"Why did you use your arms to get out of the chair?"

I told her I hadn't thought about it.

She said, "Sit down again, and then get up without using your arms."

Try as I might, it was impossible for me to do. "I guess I am just getting old," I said.

"No," she said. "You are too young for this. I would like to do a quick neurological workup."

She did a few tests of my strength and reflexes and then referred me to a neurologist who had received her training at the University of California, San Diego Medical School, where they specialize in neuromuscular diseases.

The neurologist put me through a long battery of tests, including blood work, a chest x-ray, an MRI of my entire spine, and the infamous electromyogram.

For those who have not had the pleasure, I will describe that last test. It consists of having needles inserted into your muscles, generally in your legs, arms and hands. Then you are asked to move. The needles are connected to a machine that makes a noise like radio static. Those sounds are the electrical response of your muscles and nerves as you activate them. This part of the test is only mildly unpleasant since the needles are very small diameter - like acupuncture needles. The real "fun" starts when the doctor sends electrical shocks through the wires, causing your muscles to contract in response.

At the end of the appointment, the neurologist told me she believed I had some kind of illness that was affecting both my nerves and my muscles. She said I should be prepared to have a disease that that is incurable. She also told me that she was going to refer me to her former professor who was very knowledgeable about rare muscle diseases.

Next came a long wait - nearly two months from the time I left the neurologist's office until my next appointment. In the meantime, I wondered what I could possibly have. This was before the days when you could type a few keywords into an Internet browser and get all kinds of answers; instead we had our trusty medical Encyclopedia. I looked up diseases of the nerves and muscles and only found one that seemed to make sense: amyotrophic lateral sclerosis (Lou Gehrig's Disease). The more I read about it, the more it seemed to fit all of my symptoms. ALS usually progresses rapidly, so I began to prepare for the end. I made lists of all the things I wanted to tell my children, I organized our financial records, and I allowed myself to grieve for the life I thought I would lose. I didn't tell my wife and children yet, just in case the diagnosis was not so dire.

The appointment with the UCSD neurologist finally arrived. He came into the examining room followed by several neurology students, standard practice for a teaching hospital. He asked me to stand and walk over to shake his hand. When I did, he turned to the students. "I believe I have reached the point where I can diagnose this particular illness just by watching a patient's gait," he said. "I am quite certain that this man has inclusion body myositis - IBM."

He spent another few minutes with me and explained that the only way to diagnose IBM with more certainty was to do a muscle biopsy. He also said there was no treatment available that had been shown to be of benefit, although some doctors recommended trying drugs intended to suppress the immune system since they were effective on polymyositis, a related disease. I asked if they were of any help to IBM and he said they were not, as far as he knew. I also asked if they had side effects and he said yes, they did. So why would I want to take them? Once again he turned to his students. "This is a good example of where you may do a patient more harm than good by trying to treat him."

Before he left, the doctor gave me a newsletter from The Myositis Association along with the phone number of the coordinator of a local support group for all forms of myositis. These were helpful but I wish I had asked more questions. My symptoms went back 10 years, wouldn't that affect my prognosis? Were there any long-term studies available?

A few weeks later I was back at UCSD, where the chief of neurosurgery performed a muscle biopsy. The skin is given a local anesthetic and a scalpel is used to make about a 2-inch incision. The muscle sample is removed for later analysis under an electron microscope. They are looking for telltale rimmed vacuoles and inclusion bodies. Whether they find them or not can depend on the location of the sample. Some people may need to have the biopsy repeated.

When my biopsy result came back, it was "Consistent with inclusion body myositis." So now I knew what I had, but no idea what I really faced. The doctors assured me that this disease was slow moving and did not directly affect my ability to breathe, so I would likely die of something altogether different. What they did not tell me then, was that this slow-moving disease had been working on me for a long time and its effects would soon become much more dramatic. I have since learned that IBM can affect your ability to breathe, information that wasn't available when I was diagnosed.

# Hooray, I Have Inclusion Body Myositis

This will sound irrational, but I was almost giddy following the confirmation of my diagnosis. During the months preceding I had quietly convinced myself that I only had a couple of years to live, so when they told me that it was a slowly progressive disease, I thought, "How wonderful!" During the first few years after I had been diagnosed, friends, neighbors and family members would remark on how good-natured I appeared considering my illness. Well if any of them are reading this, now they know the truth. Of course if things had happened in the opposite order, my reaction would have been quite different I am sure.

My optimism was also a result of the lack of information about inclusion body myositis. Polymyositis, a treatable disease, had been around for quite a while. Doctors were learning that many people with polymyositis who didn't respond to treatment actually had inclusion body myositis.

Medical books either ignored IBM or allocated just a few lines of information. There were no long-term studies that showed what one should expect. Most of what I read back then said that IBM might *eventually* lead to the need for an assistive mobility device of some kind. So I assumed that I could just go about my regular life for many years and perhaps when I was old and feeble, I would need a walker or maybe a scooter.

I have since learned that progressive muscular illness should never be taken lightly. Even if it does not shorten your life, it may cause significant changes in the way you live.

Today if you are diagnosed with inclusion body myositis, with a little research you can have a fairly good idea of what may lie ahead. In fact, at the end of this book there is a chapter titled "Timeline of Disability," which lists each of my losses of physical function - and the adaptive measures I was forced to take - in chronological order. I would gladly have paid a thousand times the price of this book to have that information when I was first diagnosed.

Now, as they say in many ads, "Your results may vary." Not everyone experiences the same kinds of disabilities or at the same rate. If you have a different form of progressive muscular illness, it may not even affect the same muscle groups and it may be treatable. At the time of this writing, there are some promising studies evaluating possible treatments for inclusion body myositis, described in more detail later. This information is changing rapidly. The best way to keep informed about treatments and trials is to keep checking the National Institutes of Health website.

# Maybe We Should Move

When I returned to the neurologist at my local clinic to discuss my results, I half-jokingly said, "Maybe we should move to a single-story home."

She did not laugh. Instead she said, "That might be a good idea." I felt a chill pass through my body. For the first time I wondered if I really needed to take this disease seriously.

But then I thought, "That's silly. I can still walk, even jog a little. I am playing some golf and tennis. So what if all of our bedrooms are on the second floor, up a long flight of stairs?"

That was in the spring of 1996. I was 55 years old (the statistical average for new diagnoses of IBM). By the end of the year, I had fallen down that long flight of stairs twice, had stopped playing golf and had given up tennis after a bad fall on the court.

Throughout this time, my wife had been very supportive. When I mentioned what the doctor said about moving, she immediately contacted a real estate agent. I know this must have been terribly hard for her, as she loved our home. It was where we had raised our daughters and hosted dozens of parties and family gatherings. We expected to live there for many more years. But one thing I have learned through this journey with IBM is that it has a way of changing your plans. I've also learned there is a tendency for people with progressive muscle disease to make small changes when bigger ones are called for.

This is an important point. If you're like most people, you will want to make the smallest, least disruptive, least expensive lifestyle modification possible to accommodate your new situation. But the truth is, in the long run this may be the most disruptive and expensive way to go. Your disease may not progress as far as mine or as quickly. However, the odds are pretty good that you're going to need to make some major accommodations in the years that follow.

When we looked for our next home, we focused our attention on finding a home with a ground-floor master bedroom, so I wouldn't have to climb stairs on a daily basis. This is one example where planning ahead would have saved us time and money. There are so many other things we could have considered. What if I ended up in a wheelchair? How would that change the accommodations we needed? We could have considered the safety issues. What if there was a problem in one of the rooms and I was the only one home? Wouldn't it be a good idea that I might be able to get into the garage when I was using a wheelchair? Overlooking those considerations wound up costing us tens of thousands of dollars, because our first choice of a home was unsuitable a few years later after my illness had progressed. Selling one home and buying another is very expensive – and when renovation is needed to make the home accessible, the costs increase dramatically.

If someone had handed me this book back in early 1997, we would have looked for a home that was all on one floor, that didn't have tiny cramped hallways with multiple doors next to each other, that didn't have a sunken living room, and had a kitchen large enough to be easily modified for a wheelchair-using chef.

If you're about to launch a search for more accessible housing, I suggest you cut to the chase. Look for a house that is handicap accessible, and that doesn't simply mean one that has no steps leading to the front door. Following are some suggestions. (By all means do your own research to confirm local building codes and requirements.)

The inside of the house should all be on one level, and there should be no steps or at least no more than one step (which you will need to replace with a ramp).

The front entry must be wide enough for a wheelchair, even if the rider has poor vision. This means a standard 36-inch door. If the entry has double doors, make sure each is 36 inches. Otherwise you will be struggling to get both of them opened and closed several times a day. Also be sure there is at least one other exterior door a wheelchair could get through in an emergency.

Is there room to load and unload a ramp-equipped van in the driveway or garage? If the only choice is to unload from the street, remember that the parking spaces might be taken.

Interior hallways should be at least 4 feet wide. The door to any room that you want to enter needs to be wide enough for a wheelchair to pass through. You can use special "swing-away" hinges that gain an extra 2 inches off the standard door opening. Even so, you will find that the standard interior 30-inch doorway is barely adequate for a wheelchair. Thirty-two-inch doors are better. (I know, I know, you aren't in a wheelchair now and you don't intend to ever be in one! This is why am writing this book. I was in that frame of mind back then, but I soon learned that a disabling illness is unpredictable.)

Floor covering can make a big difference when you are in a wheelchair. It should either be hard flooring or a tight-weave carpet with a thin pad. A soft, cushy carpet is almost impossible to push a wheelchair through and even a power chair will struggle. What's more, you will find that beautiful carpet will soon have deep ruts and irreparable damage in the areas you travel most.

Sinks with vanities look nice, but suspended sinks with plenty of room underneath are a lot easier if you're in a wheelchair.

Be sure to take a good look at the tubs and the showers unless you plan on having sponge baths in bed later on. Those new walk-in tubs are nice, provided you're walking! If tub baths are important, then eventually you'll need a lifting mechanism in the tub. A large roll-in shower is ideal, but it should have a fold-down seat too. There may be several years where you can still safely transfer to the seat for a shower.

If you spend any time on the various muscular dystrophy forums, you'll find toilets are a frequent topic of conversation. We even talk about them at our support group luncheons! Most toilets are too low for people with weak legs to rise from. Even if the home already has a "handicap height" toilet, eventually you may need to modify it with some kind of lifting device.

If the home is part of an HOA, check their clubhouse, if there is one, to be sure it is handicap accessible. If there is a pool, find out if they have a lift should you need it to get into the pool someday. This is very important because people suffering from muscle diseases often find water exercise helpful. Although the Americans with Disabilities Act requires public facilities to have pool lifts, there is a loophole for private homeowners associations, so you definitely need to ask.

If you plan on spending any time in the yard, think

about how a wheelchair could get around out there. Many homes in retirement communities use low-maintenance crushed rock in the place of sod. Wheelchairs will not roll through crushed rock. Sod is okay if it is packed down well, but if it gets muddy then you are not going to be able to get around until it dries out.

Since you aren't likely to find the "perfect" home, there are some things you can add later that won't be terribly expensive. These include a bidet for the toilet (trust me, when your hands get weak you'll know why you need this), ceiling lifts to get you from wheelchair to bed if you become so disabled that you cannot stand, swing away hinges on any doors that are difficult to get through, laminate flooring to replace carpet, and additional hardscape outside so that you can access more of your yard or garden.

If you have already moved to a home that has two stories, all may not be lost. You can install a stair lift that will carry you from one floor to the next. Just keep in mind that once you reach the other floor, you will need a mobility aid waiting for you. This could mean having a second wheelchair or scooter available.

When you're looking for an accessible home, be sure to consider public transportation availability. You may not need it at the time, but someday you will. There is an entire chapter on the subject later.

After our search, we settled on a condominium just a few miles away. It had a master bedroom on the ground floor, an office, and a loft on the top floor. The floor plan seemed ideal, since my wife - an artist - needed a studio. I could set up my office in the den on the ground floor for the time when I would no longer be going to work each day. The condo was not handicap accessible by any means, but I figured we had years before I would need to worry about accommodating a scooter or wheelchair. Of course I was completely wrong about that as numerous falls and trips to urgent care would emphatically demonstrate.

Why were changes in my abilities coming so rapidly when this was supposed to be a slow-moving disease? I returned to my neurologist and asked her that question. She explained that I had probably been suffering from IBM for at least 10 years before I was diagnosed. Even though the disease only takes away about 5% of one's strength each year, I had already lost quite a bit in my quadriceps. If I stumbled, I would not have the extra strength to catch myself. My doctor recommended I start using a walking aid as soon as possible.

At that point, I was still feeling a bit foolish about using any kind of obvious device to help me stay upright. A friend gave me a high-tech hiking stick. Using it made me feel "cool." Before long I realized it wasn't enough, so I bought another one. Walking with a single stick may look cool, but walking with two is just strange.

# Getting to Know IBM

One of the best things that happened to me during this time was attending the meetings of the San Diego Keep In Touch group sponsored by The Myositis Association (TMA). Later, when the Muscular Dystrophy Association added IBM to its list of covered diseases, MDA shared sponsorship. Through those meetings, we learned the Myositis Association held a national conference each year. There was going to be one in the fall of 1997 in Washington, DC, and we decided to go. When my wife and I entered the convention hall and saw the hundreds of people gathered, we realized that I was by no means alone. Looking around the hall, I wondered whether I truly belonged there, since many of the attendees rode scooters or wheelchairs. The day before, my wife and I – with the help of my walking stick - had hiked the length of the National Mall, twice. Was this really "my" disease? A few years later, at the Houston national conference, it would be me on a scooter reassuring other newcomers that they were in the right place.

We learned a lot about IBM at our first national conference. We learned there was still no treatment, let alone a cure, and that research was progressing very slowly since the disease was so rare. This information came from the head of muscle diseases at the National Institutes of Health, along with other nationally recognized experts in the field of neurology. During breaks and at meals we had the chance to hear about the experiences of other people with IBM.

Inclusion body myositis is just one of a large

number of "orphan" diseases that are so rare they have few resources for finding cures or treatments. If you have such a disease, you'll probably find a support group network organized by others with the same disease. You should join it to get information and make connections. It makes a huge difference when you get to know other people who are going through similar problems. I would need another book just to list all of the help I have received over the years through my friendships with members of our local support group. Anyone who has been diagnosed with a form of myositis should consider attending a national conference, and continue to participate regularly as long as your health allows it.

Much of what I have learned about the progression of IBM has been real-world information, not scientific studies or published articles, but firsthand accounts from others with the disease. I believe personal narratives (such as the one you're reading) are an important source of information you can use.

The most obvious characteristics of IBM are the weakness in the quadriceps muscles and hands. More than half of all people with inclusion body myositis also suffer from dysphagia, the inability to swallow properly, due to weak facial muscles. You will read in most articles that inclusion body myositis does not affect the ability to breathe, however, my experience has been different. I cover that in depth in a later chapter.

At that first national conference we learned that there was no agreement among the experts about the cause of inclusion body myositis. Was it an autoimmune disease? Maybe. Some thought it might be triggered by a virus or by environmental influences. They were fairly certain that it was not a hereditary illness – at least not the type I had, sporadic inclusion body myositis or sIBM. (There is a hereditary form of inclusion body myositis that is even more rare.) The classic muscular dystrophies are hereditary, which means that IBM is not usually classed with muscular dystrophy, although it has much in common with some of those diseases.

In addition to polymyositis, there are two other myositis illnesses: dermatomyositis and juvenile dermatomyositis. These forms of myositis have treatments available, but they can also be more serious if untreated. For more information about them, I recommend visiting The Myositis Association and Muscular Dystrophy Association websites. Their web addresses are in the back of this book.

As this book is being written, a lot has changed in the approach to understanding IBM. The human genome has been catalogued and researchers are looking more closely at how the behaviors of specific genes influence disease processes. It is quite likely that this research will eventually lead to some kind of treatment or even a cure. For right now, the best thing you can do is to adapt and avoid serious injury that would make it impossible for you to take advantage of a treatment or cure in the future.

# Falling and Rising

My first few years with inclusion body myositis were the most dangerous. I was still trying to live a "normal" life even though I was falling more often.

I continued to work for several years after I was diagnosed. A friend and I had started an advertising agency. Since there were only the two of us, we each took on many roles within the agency. When I was diagnosed, I assured my partner we could continue in business as always. I actually believed it. There were only two problems that would get in my way: Falling down and getting up.

There is something unique about falling when you have IBM. One moment you are upright and then you are on the floor wondering how you got there. It is as if a trap door had suddenly opened beneath you. During those first years, I fell in parking lots, car dealerships, stores, and all over our home. For me, the most upsetting falls were those where other people saw it happen. (Kind of silly, since falling with nobody around meant that I would have to stay on the ground until someone showed up.)

Worst of all were the falls in front of my clients. Advertising is all about image-building. It's difficult to convince someone that you know how to make a company look good when you're sitting on the ground waiting to be helped up.

Even if I didn't *fall* in front of a client, there was the chair problem. As the quadriceps – the big muscles on the front of your thighs that straighten out your legs to stand - grow weaker, you need two things to help them function. First, you need a place to put your hands so you can push down and use your shoulder muscles to help rise. Second, you need a higher chair so it takes less strength to get up. I could adjust my office chair high enough, but when I visited a client or took one to lunch, there could be trouble ahead. If I wound up in a seat that was too low, I would struggle while trying to hide my difficulty from my client.

If falls were so risky and embarrassing, why didn't I use a walker? I'm sure that pride had a lot to do with it. I would rather risk a broken ankle, or wrist, or skull, than tell the world I was disabled. Truth is, some clients did stop giving me work when they saw my weakness firsthand. Others were very understanding, especially those in businesses related to medicine.

Why didn't I simply call it quits? Inclusion body myositis often shows up around the age of 55, which for most people is right in the prime of their career. It's a key time to beef up retirement funds that may have been neglected earlier. That was certainly the case for my partner and me, so I was determined to keep working as long as possible. This may have been an admirable financial choice, but it came at a great personal cost. Those were the years when I was still healthy enough to travel by air, and to enjoy my family at the fullest. Looking back, I can't be positive that I would have done things differently, but I like to think so.

# Buy a Scooter, Sell a Car

After we moved into our condo, we had it adapted to suit our needs, or so we thought. I was out back doing some yard work and stepped down off the patio. The next thing I knew I went head first into a wall. That led to spending some quality time in a doctor's office as he dug pieces of stucco out of my scalp. Eventually I realized I needed more walking support, so I got a walker. I thought that would surely last me for many years to come.

It lasted just a few months. I was in our living room and the walker was wedged between two chairs. I tried to pull it free and the next thing I knew I was falling straight back with no way to stop myself. I can still remember the crashing sound inside my head when I hit the floor. Fortunately, I came out of it with only a mild concussion, but I realized I needed to be even more careful if I was going to survive.

I decided to buy a three-wheel scooter. I had purchased one for my mother when she had gone into a retirement facility, so I was not too terribly concerned about how I might look riding one. In fact, I looked forward to it when I realized it would give me a lot more range around the neighborhood and eliminate the fear of falling outside. It wouldn't do anything to help the problem indoors. That was going to have to wait, because our condo had a step at the front door, another one down into the living room, and yet another out onto the back patio.

Buying one piece of equipment always seems to lead to the need for many others. Once I had the scooter, I needed some way to haul it around with me when I drove somewhere. My car at that time was a two-door Acura

Integra coupe with a stick shift, sunroof, sports suspension and a powerful engine. That is what I was driving when I went scooter shopping. I asked the owner of the mobility dealership how I would transport my new scooter. He pointed to a used Plymouth minivan in his lot. It had a lift that swung out from the back compartment. I could hook the scooter onto it, pick it up and swing it inside. I knew he was right, but I resisted for a few days before buying the van and giving the Acura to my daughter.

I still get a little misty-eyed thinking about how I felt as she drove out of the parking lot and off to college. There would be no more racing up and down the mountain roads of San Diego County for me. But the van did open new opportunities for travel and shopping, as I could now take my "legs" along. One other important purchase I made was a folding fiberglass ramp to keep in the van. Many times we would go to a friend's house or to an event and discover there was a step or a curb in the way. With that ramp, we were prepared.

By 1999, I was finding it very treacherous to walk even a short distance within our house. The scooter was great for cruising around the neighborhood and going shopping, but it was of little use in the house, even if I could find a way to get it inside. The scooter didn't turn sharply enough to get through the narrow kitchen entrance or into the utility room. So I needed a power wheelchair to use indoors. By this time I was sufficiently disabled that I thought I could get help with the cost of the wheelchair through my health insurance. My neurologist sent me to a physiatrist, a medical doctor who specializes in physical medicine, who wrote a prescription for a power wheelchair. She also suggested that I see an orthotist for leg braces that might allow me to continue walking.

That was when I met Larry, a remarkable gentleman (and orthotist) who had lost both legs as a child. I did not know this when he walked into the room and if he had not told me, I would never have known that his legs were artificial. This was obviously someone who would provide me with the best equipment for my needs.

Larry fitted me with a pair of lightweight carbon fiber braces that went from my foot to the top of my thigh. They had special hinges at the knees. Each hinge locked when I put weight on the leg but immediately released when I raised my leg in a walking motion. The braces were not safe to use by themselves; I also needed to have a pair of forearm crutches. As time-consuming as they were to put on, I have never regretted using them. They allowed me to keep walking for several more years, although I would grow tired quickly and needed to use the wheelchair and scooter as well.

Once I overcame my initial embarrassment about being disabled, I have embraced mobility aids. They have helped me get out more, and fall less.

# Buy a Wheelchair, Remodel a House

The wheelchair was a Jazzy, made by Pride Mobility, one of the earliest models of wheelchairs designed to look a little less "medical." Today it seems amusing that I was concerned about being seen using a piece of equipment that would be so useful. Yet I frequently hear fellow sufferers declare that they will never allow themselves to be seen in a wheelchair. Maybe if they knew that, according to the 2010 census, there are 3.3 million of us in wheelchairs, they would feel a little differently. I was fortunate to have my insurance pay for about half the cost of the wheelchair and the braces. Even so, my out-of-pocket expense was several thousand dollars. But every new piece of equipment seems to have its own list of requirements, and most will cost money.

Since I intended to use my wheelchair indoors, the next issue was how to get it inside and how to maneuver it throughout the condo. There were several issues that had to be addressed. Our front walk had two steps that led to the front door. There was a large step at the back door. There was another step from the entryway down to the living room. (Why are builders still making homes with unnecessary changes of level on the ground floor? Should any of the occupants become disabled, they may find it impossible to remain in their home.) Several of the inside doors were too narrow to get through in a wheelchair, and the bathroom was an absolute nightmare with a massive concrete and tile Roman tub at one end. Up to this point I had been managing to climb over the side and take a shower, but it was very risky and one fall could have been catastrophic. Getting rid of the tub would be expensive and difficult, but it had to go. I knew this because of an experience we had on our 24th wedding anniversary the year before.

We flew into Seattle, rented a car and drove to the town of Sequim on the north shore of the Olympic Peninsula. We had been up in the area several times before and had always remarked about how it might be a great place to retire. We decided to take one last look, since I was surely going to be forced into retirement soon. After checking into Juan de Fuca cottages, we immediately headed to The Three Crabs restaurant, perhaps our favorite restaurant ever. It sat right at the shoreline near Dungeness Point, hence the name.

We had a terrific feast of Dungeness crab, mussels, clams, scallops and shrimp accompanied by a bottle of Kendall Jackson Grand Reserve Chardonnay. When we got back to our cottage, we were in the mood to celebrate. The cottage had a large raised Roman tub, not unlike the one in our condo back home. However this one was even larger and equipped with water jets. So we both jumped in. Well, that is an exaggeration; we each climbed in gingerly. When it was time to get out, my wife exited first and then I tried to climb over the side of the tub only to discover I couldn't. Now what? We were in one of seven small cottages, the manager had long since gone to bed, and a 911 call seemed excessive. So my wife dug in her heels on the side of the tub and pulled with all her might as I tried to heave myself over the edge and, after about a half-hour of struggling, I was finally free - although very sore.

Getting rid of the Roman tub back home took two days of jackhammering before it was broken up and removed. (Five years later when we sold the condo, we were still trying to get the concrete dust out of our clothes.) We replaced it with a roll-in shower that had a sloping floor covered in one-inch nonskid tile. By the way, if you build a roll-in shower or even re-tile the bathroom floor, be certain to get the genuine nonskid tiles. There are some that will seem like they have a rough surface when they are dry, but as soon as they get wet they turn into a skating rink! We were lucky to have a contractor who specialized in accessible remodeling and he knew the difference.

To get my scooter and wheelchair into the house we needed to remove the front porch and walkway and replace them with a sloping concrete ramp. Then we added a carpeted ramp connecting the entryway to the living room. Now I could at least get into the house with my wheelchair. But I still couldn't get into the bedroom. It turned out there was an easy solution for making the doors wider with those "swing away" hinges I mentioned earlier. They have an offset design that allows the full width of the door opening to be used. We installed a pair of those on the bedroom door. We also had a concrete ramp constructed at the back door so that I could get out onto the patio, and we built a breakfast bar along one side of the kitchen that was high enough for me to drive beneath it in the wheelchair. That came in handy later on when I started doing more of the cooking. The total cost of all of these modifications was about $8,000 - money well spent in my opinion, even though none of it was covered by insurance.

Many people think (hope) that health insurance will pay for the kind of home modifications required to make it handicap accessible. Most will not, except for the Veterans Administration. Medicare definitely won't, nor will they pay for a handicap accessible vehicle.

# Quit Work, Become an Artist

At the end of 1999, I was forced to stop working, which meant my partner had to retire as well. We closed the doors of the advertising agency and went our separate ways. He bought a motorhome and left on a trip around the continent with his wife. I went home and worried. How would we get by without any business income?

Then, at a Myositis Association support group meeting, one of the members suggested I apply for Social Security disability. I had never even given that a thought, but I realized it might be the answer to our dilemma. I was only 59 years old and would not be eligible for full Social Security for another six and a half years. Maybe I could get it early. I filled out all the paperwork, including giving the Social Security Administration a very detailed explanation of my condition and why it prevented me from continuing to work. Soon I received a letter instructing me to go to the local office for an evaluation by their physician.

I had been warned that it is very difficult to get approved for Social Security disability. Most people are turned down when they apply, and many find it necessary to hire an attorney. This is especially true for those with a rare disease like inclusion body myositis, since it is not common knowledge how severely people can be affected.

As luck would have it, the Social Security physician who saw me had been trained at the University of California, San Diego and knew all about IBM. As soon as she learned what I had, she approved my application. I had worked my entire life and had always contributed the maximum amount, which meant I would be receiving more than $1,500 per month. What's more, after two years I could go on Medicare, greatly reducing my health insurance premiums and giving me far better coverage. Combined with our relatively modest savings and my IRA account, we would be able to get by, we thought. Later we would learn that having a disability is far more expensive than anyone might imagine.

By the time I retired, I had given up just about every activity that had occupied me for the past 50 years. No more running, biking, golfing, tennis, fishing, hiking, camping, or playing the piano. The last few months of work had been very exhausting, so I spent several months doing almost nothing but riding my scooter around the neighborhood and surfing the Internet. Before long I was getting bored and wondering what to do next. My wife, on the other hand, was having a good time going upstairs to her studio and creating watercolor paintings. She would bring them down at the end of the day to show me what she was working on. Why not try to become an artist myself?

At first, I needed to learn some very basic things, like how to draw. My engineering education and career as a writer weren't exactly the hallmarks of a future artist, but I was stubborn and determined to learn. In the summer of 2000, we traveled to Ocean Park, WA, a small town on the Long Beach Peninsula just north of the Oregon border. My wife attended a watercolor workshop taught by a well-known artist. I spent the week cruising around the area on my scooter and doing some photography and sketching. I also got the chance to look in on some of the classes. By the end of the week, I was hooked.

My wife was a member of the San Diego Watercolor Society (SDWS) and I started attending monthly demonstrations with her. There I learned about the

"Wednesday Morning Painters," a group of artists that gathered each week at a scenic spot to set up their easels and paint. At the end of the morning, they critiqued each other's work. Some were experienced painters, but there were also beginners. Joining this group seemed a good way for me to get started.

I couldn't walk around and find different angles of a building or a body of water or a grove of trees. However, I adapted my scooter into a rolling art studio. I built a basket on the front that held my painting supplies and portable easel, and I hung an art bag over the side for watercolor paper and backing board. This arrangement gave me an advantage because I could travel long distances from our meeting point and be ready to paint when I found a scene I liked.

The first paintings were absolutely horrible, but after a few months I was creating some work worth framing and entering into the local SDWS show. About that time, the person who was in charge of the Wednesday Morning Painters group wanted to take a break and asked if I would be willing to take over. That turned out to be the beginning of a very long relationship with the Watercolor Society. The most important part of the job was to select the painting locations for each week and provide the members with a list covering the next couple of months. My engineering mentality kicked in and I thought, "Database!" I gathered all of the information about every site that the group had visited and put it into a database. Then I went out in my van and surveyed several other spots and added them to the list. I was able to create a full year of weekly painting with no repeats. Of course being in San Diego with good weather most of the year and 70 miles of scenic coastline made that less of a challenge.

My list of locations is still on the Internet, now embellished with photographs, maps and paintings. You can see it by visiting http://shirkstudios.com/ShirkStudiosPleinAir.htm.

After a couple of years, I was invited to join the SDWS Board of Directors as Membership Chairman. Once again I used my computer experience to create an improved database of their 750 members. This led to revamping their website to become interactive so that members could update their own information, pay bills, and even enter paintings into shows. In 2006, I was elected President of the group. My paintings were improving and eventually would be shown in major competitions throughout the west and purchased by collectors around the country.

As I look back on the 10-year journey I had with watercolor and the San Diego Watercolor Society, I realize how lucky I was to have such a passion at that time of my life. I made new friends, gave my life added purpose, and made a contribution to the community. I was very busy during that time, but always seemed to have a positive outlook. Now I am no longer able to pick up a brush, let alone create a work of art. The good news is that voice recognition has allowed me to return to my original love of writing.

# Get Out of Town

Once I retired, we began to travel more - but not as much as we should have. Over the space of six years, we took six trips along the Pacific Coast plus one to the Grand Canyon and another to Texas. We also took two trips that were especially noteworthy because of the difficulties we encountered.

Each year, the logistics of travel became more complicated. For our first trips, we only needed to put my scooter in the back of the van, along with a bathroom booster seat and my BiPAP breathing machine (used during sleep). I was still very comfortable with driving. If motel rooms had challenging layouts, my scooter was strong enough to move furniture quite well. Of course every time we stopped, I had to get out of the driver's seat, hang onto the side of the car and work my way around to the back where I could use the lift to unload the scooter and sit down. All went well until we went to Las Vegas.

The drive from San Diego to Las Vegas is not especially scenic. In fact, it is downright boring for much of the way. This is one reason we had always avoided going there. Besides, we were not gamblers, and we could see shows in San Diego. But then we heard about a new resort that had opened and we decided to take the drive.

We were still 30 miles outside the city when we crested a rise and an enormous golden building loomed above the desert. A half hour later we were at the end of a long line of cars waiting to unload at the front entrance. One of the attendants noticed our handicap placard and motioned for us to move to another line that was almost empty. But when we got there, another attendant yelled at us for cutting in line and refused to help unload our luggage.

I got out of the van and cautiously worked my way around to unload my scooter. The hotel's entry was paved with odd-shaped cobblestones, and I only made it about halfway before I fell. I could feel a sharp pain in my ankle, but I was determined to get my scooter and our luggage out of the van, so I struggled upright, unloaded the scooter and luggage and rolled into the lobby.

At the front desk, I reminded the clerk that we had reserved a handicap accessible room. I was assured we had been assigned one. However, when we opened the door to the room it was too crowded with furniture for the scooter to get in and the bathroom had a regular tub and a low toilet. The room was obviously not handicap accessible. I returned to the front desk and the clerk sent me to another room. It was no better than the first. This time I called the desk and they sent someone up to see what was wrong.

When I explained that we were supposed to have a handicap accessible room, the employee pointed to a light over the doorway and said that when our phone rang the light would flash – so this was their idea of handicap accessible? It would have been funny if I had not been in so much pain from my earlier fall. After another hour of dealing with people who had no concept of physical disability, we wound up in a room where I could lie down on the bed and rest my foot. As soon as I removed my shoe and sock, we could see the foot was badly swollen and turning a deep shade of purple.

Another call to the lobby brought up the hotel doctor, who said it was a mild sprain and not to worry about it.

After three miserable days in Las Vegas, we drove home where my doctor x-rayed my foot and discovered it was broken.

Obviously, I wrote a nasty letter to the hotel. They sent us a coupon good for 50 percent off our next visit. I am happy to report we never used that coupon.

Our next trip was to a resort in Sedona, AZ. It was a very expensive but beautiful place and we had paid for a room with a view of the famous red rocks. We had also explained our need for a handicap accessible room. They knew exactly what we meant and told me they had two of those rooms. They were both in the basement next to utility areas and had an unobstructed view of the hotel dumpsters. For this they were charging nearly $300 per night.

To add insult to injury, when I asked for some ice, they told me it was self-serve and directed me down the hall. When I got to the ice machine, it was on a high pedestal completely out of reach of anyone in a wheelchair.

Fortunately, these were isolated incidents and seemed to happen only when we ventured inland. As long as we traveled along the Pacific Coast, we found everyone to be very accommodating of the disabled.

I fell more than once on our travels, usually when I was walking around the side of the van or when I was getting the scooter out of the rear compartment. We travelled that way for the next three years, until I finally hit my head enough times to knock some sense into me. In 2004 we bought a van with a ramp and transfer seat.

Like most of the purchases we made to improve my safety and mobility, I soon wondered how I ever got along without it. I just lowered the ramp and drove right in. After parking the scooter behind the front seats, I used a switch to bring the driver's seat back to me. Once I slid onto the seat it turned and brought me to the front in driving position. This completely eliminated the dangerous process of trying to walk around to the back of the van. However, it did mean that I needed to have sufficient strength to slide from the scooter onto the van seat. I was able to do that for several more years.

I still feel guilty that we didn't travel more - and farther. I didn't feel confident in my ability to haul my equipment onto an airplane. That took a lot of possible destinations out of the picture. My wife had always wanted to go to New York or to Europe, but it just did not seem feasible. If I had known how few years she had left, I would have found a way, probably by hiring a traveling companion to help us out. Not only could I have given my wife the experiences she craved, I would have been building a larger storehouse of memories for later years.

Our last trip was to Monterey, CA for our 30th wedding anniversary. This was appropriate, since Monterey had been part of our honeymoon trip and a favorite destination throughout our married lives. As I look at the pictures from that last journey, I can see the sadness in my wife's eyes. She realized we were not going to be able to take trips like that anymore.

# The Inventor I Always Wanted to Be

When I was young, I always thought I would be a scientist. I even attended three years of engineering school at Purdue University with that in mind. I dropped out after my junior year and from then on my only exposure to engineering was reading Popular Science magazine. Then along came inclusion body myositis and, as they say, necessity is the mother of invention. I had a lot of necessity.

In 2005, my strength went downhill rapidly. I was losing much of the muscle in my arms and hands. That is when I began making adaptive devices to help me cope.

I discovered that a dowel rod along with some threaded plastic covered hooks could produce a number of useful tools. The one I used the most was simply a short length of 3/4-inch diameter dowel with a plant hook screwed into the middle of it. (You can find plant hooks at any of the big box home improvement stores. They have large threads at one end and a plastic-covered hook at the other.) I could use this to open our refrigerator, drawers, and the door handles of our van. When others in our support group saw my hooks, they all wanted them. Someone volunteered to make several hundred that were used to raise funds at the next national conference of The Myositis Association.

I made other kinds of aids using a 2-foot length of dowel with various hooks and brackets screwed into the ends. These were used for dressing, pulling doors shut, getting stuff out from under a bed or the back of a cabinet, etc. Of course I bought reachers in copious quantities, mainly trying to find one that worked well. Most reachers depend on squeezing them with your fingers to bring the jaws together. It may not work if you have weak fingers. I eventually found one called an "ergonomic reacher" online. It had a smaller handle that fit inside the palm of my hand, where I did have some strength left. I can still use that kind of reacher today.

I also needed a way to get out of an easy chair. I was using my Jazzy wheelchair inside the house, but it didn't have a good enough seat to remain in all day. We purchased a power-lift recliner and I have never enjoyed sitting anywhere so much in my life. It had a motorized seat that lifted up and pushed forward. That part was a little scary since I could easily have been pushed too far and toppled over face first. There are now other models that just lift straight up which would be safer in my opinion.

I spent hours browsing the aisles of stores looking for gadgets to help me pick things up, hold them, or work around the house. Things that helped were lithium-ion powered screwdrivers, mini-vacuums, spring-loaded needle-nose pliers, and all sorts of little clamps. I found other items online. Those included the One-Touch can opener and jar opener (you can see them in action on my Life Disabled blog site) two battery-powered wine cork removers (we wore out the first one), a lemonade maker that juiced and stirred at the same time (life gave us lots of lemons), and huge quantities of hook-and-loop material – more commonly known by the brand name Velcro.

I could probably write an entire book on the subject of hook-and-loop. My wheelchair is covered with the stuff, as is my hospital bed. I've replaced most of the zippers and buttons in my life with strips of hook-and-loop material.

I simply could not find many of the things that I felt I needed, so I would make them. I was becoming too weak to work with full-size power tools. In fact the last time I tried, I watched helplessly as a spinning drill bit passed through my arm. But perhaps I could sew things together!

Online, I found a sewing machine that was perfect for my limited dexterity. It was operated by pushbuttons, with no need for a foot pedal. The controls were up front and easy for me to use. My first project was a belly bag to wear when I was in my wheelchair. It had a cloth belt and marine vinyl pockets that held my wallet, cell phone, miscellaneous tools, a hand hook, car keys and a Travel John. (The Travel John is a portable urinal that instantly turns liquid waste into a biodegradable solid which can be tossed into any trashcan.) The belt did not go around my waist; I couldn't reach my back. Instead it attached to the sides of my wheelchair. This first project worked so well I still wear it. I also sewed special aprons to wear in the wheelchair. (Don't even think about wearing a regular apron with those long dangling ties and a loop around your neck!)

You can see most of my tools and sewing projects on my blog.

# What Are the Odds?

During the early part of 2005, we realized something must be seriously wrong with Beth. She was too unsteady to walk without help – we even bought her a small scooter to help her get around. She was sleeping 12 hours a day and yet she would be exhausted as soon as she got up. We wondered if it was possible that she, too, had some form of muscle disease. What would be the odds of that? It was so unlikely that her doctor didn't take us seriously, but having received the same kind of response myself at first, I pressed the issue. That started us down a long trail of lab tests, CT scans and MRIs in search of a diagnosis or explanation for her symptoms. After the doctors ruled out the more common causes of weakness and fatigue, a neurologist told us that my wife had ALS – the same disease I thought I had back in 1996. He said that, based on her weakness and how long she had been having symptoms, she probably had no more than two or three years to live.

That diagnosis was quickly followed by visits from breathing therapists, physical therapists, and worst of all, a social worker. I say worst of all, because he advised us that our finances would not last long enough for my wife's treatment and our only hope was to dispose of our assets as quickly as possible to get qualified for Medi-Cal. I began that process by purchasing a very expensive wheelchair that I knew I would need someday but not yet. We started to think of other ways we could spend our modest savings.

Before we spent any more, we took Beth to the ALS clinic for a confirmed diagnosis so she would qualify for their assistance. We saw one of the nation's leading experts in ALS who repeated several neurological tests and came to a different conclusion.

"I've shown these results to several of my colleagues," he said, "and we agreed it seems unlikely you have ALS."

We looked at each other, unable to hide our excitement at the news.

"Before you get too enthusiastic," he said, "it's almost certain that you have some form of neuromuscular disease, and it is likely to be untreatable."

"But it might not be as rapidly progressive?"

"That's right," he said. "We recommend that you return to your neurologist and have more testing done." He handed us a list of suggested tests.

Armed with this new information, we went back to the doctor who had first diagnosed my wife. That meeting did not go so well.

As soon as we told him what we had learned at the ALS clinic and handed him the list of tests they suggested, he shook his head. "You really shouldn't go around to different doctors looking for a better diagnosis," he said. "I have much more experience at seeing patients than they do, and I am positive that my diagnosis is correct. Just go home and make the needed arrangements to deal with your illness."

He then ushered us out of his office.

Once again we were crushed, but we weren't ready to give up. The MDA doctor who had confirmed my diagnosis was also an expert in many other muscle illnesses, so I took Beth to see him. That doctor repeated the EMG (you know, the needles, the electric shocks) and then reassured us that my wife did not have ALS and that she probably had a completely different illness, myotonic muscular dystrophy, which could be confirmed by genetic testing.

After a few weeks we got the results. Myotonic dystrophy (also referred to as MMD) can be diagnosed by counting the number of times a particular sequence of proteins is repeated on the DMPK gene. Anything up to about 35 repeats is normal. Beth had 212 repeats, which meant she definitely had the illness.

That disease came with its own difficult baggage. It is inherited, autosomal dominant, which means that either Beth's mother or father must have had myotonic dystrophy. Since both were deceased, we couldn't know for certain which one passed the illness along to Beth. It would have been good to know this so we could have warned other members of her family. Also, we knew that each of our daughters had a 50 percent chance of having the disease. Neither had signs of the disease but symptoms don't necessarily show up until a person is later in life. The only way to know for certain was through genetic testing. Because our daughters were at the age where they would want to start families it was important they be tested immediately. Myotonic dystrophy has a congenital form that can produce life-threatening symptoms in newborns. For once, we beat the odds and neither have the illness. There was only a one in four chance of them both escaping MMD.

While we are on the subject of odds, my illness, inclusion body myositis, affects about one in every 100,000 people. Beth had just been diagnosed with an illness that affects one in every 8,000 people. The odds of the two of us having these rare diseases were one in 800 million. We had a better chance of winning several lotteries than we did of having these two rare diseases.

# Getting to Know Myotonic Dystrophy

My wife had a disease that was far more complicated than mine. IBM almost exclusively affects the muscles. Myotonic dystrophy is a systemic illness and its effects show up nearly everywhere in the body. Looking back, I know that Beth's primary care doctor never understood the far-reaching effects of her illness. Otherwise, she might have inquired more about my wife's earlier years.

We were told that, because Beth's symptoms developed relatively late in life, she had a mild case of the disease. But the doctors were just looking at the muscle weakness. Considering all of the various ways myotonic dystrophy can manifest, it was clear she had been affected from a much earlier age. You can see a diagram of systems affected on Beth's memorial website at http://beth.shirkstudios.com.

Some of these symptoms, such as digestive problems or reduced ability to focus on daily activities, are so common they could be easily attributed to other causes. But others are more specific and I wish we had done a better job of putting the pieces of the puzzle together.

For example, myotonic dystrophy causes difficulty in childbirth. Despite going through Lamaze class, being in excellent physical condition, and being very motivated to deliver our first child naturally, Beth had many hours of unproductive labor before the doctors were forced to deliver our first daughter by cesarean section. That happened when she was age 29, so it was likely the disease was having its effect at that time. She also had difficulty running. This was caused by an abnormal gait that caused her foot to slam down on the pavement. Such a gait is described in medical literature as being an indicator of myotonic dystrophy.

People with myotonic dystrophy can have life-threatening reactions to anesthesia. That happened to Beth before we learned to warn the anesthesiologist in advance.

Early onset cataracts are another symptom that is so well connected with myotonic dystrophy, ophthalmologists are told to be on the lookout for it. In hindsight, we realized it was why she had been forced to have cataract surgery at a relatively young age, yet no doctor caring for her made the connection.

The bottom line is that her symptoms had been present at least since her late 20s and quite likely earlier than that. If her doctors had figured that out, they wouldn't have considered her case to be mild at all and would have realized that she needed very aggressive treatment for the life-threatening symptoms that can emerge from myotonic dystrophy. One of those is cardiac arrhythmia, as we would learn.

# The Move We Should Have Made

Beth was not going to get better. My weakness was going to grow worse. It was time to leave our condominium. Beth was the only one using the upstairs loft, for her art studio, and she was having trouble making the climb and often falling on the way down. For several years, I had been able to get up there by climbing on my hands and knees, but no longer. This left us extremely vulnerable in case a fire broke out upstairs, since neither of us could do anything about it. We went on a search for a single-level home in a nearby retirement neighborhood. This would be the second move that we had been forced to make because of illness, but it wouldn't be the last.

In the process of looking for our next home, I learned that a "senior" neighborhood (restricted to residents age 55 and older) might be less handicap-friendly than other parts of town. This is definitely true of the Seven Oaks region of Rancho Bernardo. The development was built in the 1960s and was advertised with the slogan "The 52 Week Vacation." It was clearly targeted at people of retirement age. Even so, most of the homes were built with narrow doorways and halls and ridiculously tiny bathrooms. When the realtor was taking us around, there were many houses that we couldn't even get inside to see. Almost none of the intersections had curb cuts. I found several places where a person in a wheelchair might have to backtrack several hundred feet after reaching a dead-end at a very high curb. In addition, the sidewalks were interrupted every 60 feet by driveways with such a steep slope they could tip over a wheelchair or scooter. I seldom used a sidewalk during the years we lived in Seven Oaks. I just drove my wheelchair down the street and accepted the glares from passing motorists.

After weeks of searching, we found a home that someone else had modified to make wheelchair-friendly and it was perfect for the two of us. It had begun as a very small two-bedroom house, but three major remodels added a large family room we could use for a studio, and an even larger master bedroom with plenty of room for two hospital beds and two wheelchairs. There was enough room left over to expand the master bathroom, making it fully accessible.

The previous owners had widened the halls and doorways so that no door was less than 32 inches. This is such an important feature I don't know why there aren't building codes requiring it for all homes. After all, talk to almost anyone who has bought their "dream home" and they will tell you they plan on living there forever. Most of them will eventually learn that the only way to stay is with significant renovations as they age, including adding ramps, stair lifts or elevators, moving walls and widening doorways and halls. I think Universal Housing Design is way overdue in most states.

We had a beautiful view to the north and perfect light into the studio. We thought we would spend the rest of our days happily painting together and enjoying the view. That was May of 2006. We would have to leave in May of 2012. By that time, neither of us could paint. I was too weak to raise a brush. Beth was legally blind and couldn't even enjoy the view she loved so much. But during the years in between, we really did have a wonderful time painting during the day and enjoying a drink by the large north-facing window in the evening.

Despite the ideal layout of the house, we spent a lot

of money making it fully accessible. The two problem areas were the bathrooms and the yard. The master bathroom was a typical 1960s design with barely enough room for a toilet and a small shower stall. I was too weak to take a shower while standing. I needed a much larger area where I could sit on a bench. I had also lost so much finger strength that personal hygiene was a challenge, so I needed room for a toilet with a bidet. The improvements we made are difficult to describe in words, but there is a diagram on my Life Disabled blog that pretty well explains it. The changes cost about $15,000.

For the other bathroom, which Beth was to use, we needed to do something about the tub. Although she could manage to get into a bathtub, it was a risky process for her to get back out. We bought a bathtub lift that had a battery driven motor to raise the seat so Beth could easily sit down and be lowered to the floor of the tub. After bathing, the seat would bring her back up, provided we remembered to charge the battery. (Did we ever forget? Oh yes!)

During these years, it was easy to fool ourselves into believing we could live like this indefinitely. Beth had her own wheelchair, so she was much less likely to fall, and I had completely given up walking. However I was beginning to have more trouble with simply standing. To get dressed in the morning, I would lean against a wall while Beth pulled up my pants. To get into bed, I used a sliding board and pushed myself from the wheelchair onto the bed. Then I would use a sling made out of shelf liner to pull my right leg the rest of the way onto the bed. This was getting to be more and more difficult.

Just before things got so hard, I received some help from an unexpected source. The leader of our support group, a wonderful man named Charlie Harber, had died of aspiration pneumonia, a condition that frequently leads to the end for people with inclusion body myositis. His wife asked if anyone needed the ceiling lift they had been using to transfer him. I wasn't convinced that I needed it yet but I told her I would love to have it. I also purchased another ceiling lift. It was a long distance from my bed to the master bathroom and I would need an extremely long track. With two lifts, I could have one over my bed and one in the bathroom. Add up some more expenses, about $5,000, to inclusion body myositis. I would learn I couldn't have made a more important investment.

You might not think the outside of the house would be of concern, but in our neighborhood, the emphasis was on low-maintenance yards. That meant crushed rock instead of grass. Our very first day in the new house, I decided to explore the backyard and discovered an important fact: wheelchairs do not roll on crushed rock. Instead, they dig themselves in deeper and deeper until they are hopelessly stuck. That's how I announced my presence to the neighborhood, sitting in a wheelchair buried up to the fenders, yelling for help.

That evening I laid out a plan of sidewalks that would take me to all the important areas of the yard. This included the fruit trees, the vegetable garden (actually three half wine barrels so I could reach the plants from the wheelchair), the irrigation system, the hedges and rose bushes, the air conditioner, the electrical box, and hose connections. Altogether we added 200 linear feet of sidewalk plus about 500 square feet of patio. We also widened the concrete driveway. It needed to be 16 feet across, to make room for the van with the ramp lowered and still have clearance for me to maneuver the wheelchair onto the ramp. Although we had a one-and-one-half car garage, it was about 3 feet too narrow for lowering the ramp, so we had to use the driveway for getting the wheelchair into and out of the van. The concrete and labor were another $6,000.

# Attack of the Flesh-Eating Freezer

About three years after we moved into the house, I had ended my volunteer service for the San Diego Watercolor Society. I was also painting less, which left me with more time on my hands. I spent a lot of that time trying to solve the problems inclusion body myositis was tossing my way. One of those problems might seem silly, unless you spend all of your time in a wheelchair. It turns out that ordinary pants are not made for people who are going to sit from the time they get up until the time they go to bed. The waistband is too high in the front and too low in the back. Both of those issues cause discomfort and occasionally embarrassment.

Through the Internet, I discovered a company called USA Jeans that made pants designed for people who sat all day - especially people in wheelchairs. These pants had a fuller seat, a lower front, a higher back, and no seams running across the sitting area. (Seams can cause welts and pressure sores.) As soon as I bought one pair of those pants and tried them on, I ordered more. I have bought close to 20 pairs by now. It is funny how such a little thing can make such a huge difference in your feeling of well-being.

If I had been paying closer attention to my legs and feet, I would have noticed that they were getting larger. Not stronger, but larger. When you have a disease that prevents using your legs, it interferes with your body's ability to pump blood and lymph back toward the heart. This is a process that goes on constantly without us noticing it, unless it stops. Then you notice it big time! The condition is called edema. It showed up in my feet first, which meant that my shoe size kept increasing. I would stalk the aisles of discount stores looking for the largest possible tennis shoes. When even a size 15 was too small, it was time for action.

This launched one of the most bizarre episodes of my adaptation career. I decided to sew my own foot coverings. By the time I was finished, I had made enough different designs to fill two large laundry baskets and, eventually, one very large trashcan. Not only did the foot coverings need to be large enough to go over my grotesquely swollen feet, I needed some way to pull them on since I was no longer able to reach down that far with my hands. I also needed a way to fasten them so they wouldn't fall off. If you go to my Life Disabled YouTube page, you will find a video where I demonstrate all of these failed attempts. It is good for a laugh but not much else.

The final design I settled upon was more like a bag with straps attached. I used the straps to pull the bags over my feet and then I wrapped them around my calves and used Velcro to secure them. Although these "shoes" covered my feet, they couldn't hide the swelling that was now all the way up to my knees. My lower legs were as large as the average person's upper legs, and they were ugly shades of red. Most alarming of all was when I would accidentally poke one of my legs with a sharp object. Suddenly the room would resemble a crime scene, covered in puddles of blood.

How could things get much worse? All it took was a trip to the grocery store. I was in the freezer department, loading my grocery bag with a huge stack of frozen dinners (on sale) when the bag slipped off my lap and fell toward the floor. One of the handles was wrapped around my wheelchair's joystick. The wheelchair immediately charged forward, ramming my shin into the freezer door. Frantically I pulled the joystick back, but the bag was too heavy for my weak fingers and once again I lurched into the freezer door. This happened three times until finally the freezer door gave up and fell off. By this time there was a hole in my leg all the way to the bone and I was on my way to the doctor.

The doctor referred me to a local hospital's wound care clinic where they scolded me about the condition of my legs and punished me for three months. Every other day I would come in and they would scrape out stuff from my wound, repackage it with a variety of materials and then wrap both of my legs from my toes to my knees with compression bandages. This was very painful but they assured me it was the only way the wound would heal because of the severe swelling.

Once that was over, you probably think I started wearing compression hose every day. You obviously don't know me that well. I couldn't put on the compression hose by myself and I didn't want to hire someone to put them on. Instead, I sewed some additional garments that reached from my shorts to the top of my "shoes" so that no one needed to look at my legs. I was covering up a serious issue in the name of saving money. It would end up costing me.

# Take That Bus and Shove It

Despite all of the challenges, I would say the years from when we first moved into the Seven Oaks home until early 2010 were some of the most enjoyable of our married lives. Though we could not travel anymore, we had grown children who came to visit us. We also bought a 50-inch, flat-screen plasma TV and watched a lot of travel and cooking shows. After watching the movie *Julie and Julia* I was so inspired that I started cooking some of Julia Child's recipes myself. We had boef bourguignon and coq au vin that turned out quite well. The kitchen was well designed for wheelchairs, so I tried to become a serious cook. I bought a complete set of very heavy multilayer pots and pans and some excellent chef's knives. Talk about somebody needing a reality check! I had a relentlessly progressive muscle disease, yet I bought hundreds of dollars worth of very heavy pots and pans, plus dangerous knives I would soon be unable to hold. My only excuse is that I did get a lot of pleasure during the 18 months I was able to use them.

Besides cooking, I enjoyed shopping. I would drive my wheelchair into the van and head to the grocery store, being especially careful around the frozen food department.

Beth continued to paint, and she did very well in competitions, including several First Place awards in shows for disabled painters. She also was accepted twice into the prestigious San Diego Watercolor Society International Exhibition.

Once again I learned that "slowly progressive" diseases are not all that slow, especially in the way they affect your daily life. In 2010, I was having more problems using the hand controls on my van. I couldn't turn the steering wheel very easily, and braking was a huge issue. This was all brought to a head when Beth was diagnosed with breast cancer that fall. (No, she certainly didn't need another illness to deal with, but she got one anyway.) Fortunately, her cancer was caught fairly early, Stage I, so her treatment consisted of a lumpectomy followed by seven weeks of daily radiation therapy. The radiation facility was 20 miles away, which meant that every day she had to be driven a total of 40 miles. Although many of our friends pitched in to help, I still wound up making more than a dozen round trips. Each one became more frightening than the last because I was having more trouble controlling the van.

The van's hand controls relied on strength in the triceps of my left arm to push the brake lever. I was finding that more and more difficult to do, since the disease was reducing my upper body strength. The van had power steering but turning a corner was becoming an adventure.

I went to the mobility dealer that had provided me with the van and its hand controls, and asked if they could do anything to help. They put in a different steering system and more braking assistance. Once again I could turn the wheel and put on the brakes. I thought I was all set. That lasted about four or five months.

We were returning home from an appointment. I turned into our driveway and tried to slow down. No matter how hard I pushed the brake lever, the van kept moving. The front of our house had an overhang supported by 6-inch posts. I watched in horror as one of the posts came closer and closer. I managed to stop the van ... about one foot too late. The post was knocked off its foundation and that side of the overhang was now overhanging much lower. Fortunately a helpful neighbor saw what had happened and used a floor jack to lift up the post and replace it on its foundation. I realized this meant the end of my driving career.

I could have purchased a van that was controlled with the joystick and I might still be driving today. Once again, money was the deciding factor. A "drive by wire" vehicle costs about $100,000. I could not find any way to justify such an expense.

That summer, we got by okay, using our wheelchairs to get around the Rancho Bernardo area. If we had to go a longer distance, we could ask a neighbor or my daughter to drive us. But then came a winter with cold winds and rain. A simple one-mile journey to Beth's hairdresser became a trial of grit from which we would return looking like drowned rats. Why didn't we take the bus? Glad you asked, because this gives me the chance to rant about one of my favorite subjects, the lack of decent transportation services for the disabled.

Since our doctor appointments were several miles away, well out of the range of Beth's wheelchair, we had to use the bus. This is when we learned how far it was to the nearest stop. Let me rephrase that. This is when we learned how far it was to the nearest bus stop *that was wheelchair accessible*. It turned out that most of the nearby bus stops didn't have enough room to pick up a wheelchair.

Here's how it worked: The bus would pull up to the stop, and the driver would get up, walk to the rear of the bus, ask passengers in the wheelchair area to move, fold the seats out of the way, attach restraining straps to the floor, and release the safety catch on the ramp. Then the driver would walk around to the side of the bus near the back and lower a platform onto the sidewalk. The drivers were trained to be polite, but you could tell it took all of their self-control not to let you know just how much you were messing up their day. It was then your job to maneuver your wheelchair onto the platform to be lifted up to the floor level of the bus. This required a sidewalk that was wider than normal and the closest place with enough room was more than a half-mile away.

By this time Beth's eyesight was very poor, and it was a huge challenge for her to get lined up properly onto the ramp. Furthermore, she couldn't find her way around once she got off the bus. The real problem was that the bus could only take one wheelchair the size of ours at a time. So I would have to drive my wheelchair to wherever they were going to drop her off and try to meet her before she got lost. These trips became a big part of our life together for the next year.

There was also MTS Access. This was a service operated by San Diego Transit, where they would have the bus come to your home and pick you up to take you to an appointment. That might sound like an ideal solution. Let me change your mind.

Here is how the system actually works: Say you have an appointment at a medical facility four miles away at 10 a.m. The bus company tells you to allow up to two hours to reach your destination, because they will be transporting other passengers along the way. That means you need to be on the bus by 8 a.m. But you cannot simply schedule an appointment that easily. The bus company also tells you they will attempt to schedule your pickup within one hour of the time you request. So that means you must request a pickup at 7 a.m. to be assured of being picked up by 8 a.m. It is the same process coming back. However, you need to schedule your return trip taking into account the possible waiting time you may have at the doctor's office.

If you're still following along, you will see that for a simple 10 a.m. doctor visit, we needed to leave as early as 7 and expect to be home sometime in the mid-afternoon, all to travel a total of eight miles round-trip.

Now that I am alone, I could go back to using the regularly scheduled bus routes. However there is a catch. Remember when I described the process that included the bus driver moving the passengers to make room for the wheelchair? The bus company has a policy that the passengers have priority in that case and if they don't want to move, the driver must tell the wheelchair user to wait for the next bus. That has happened to me more than once, leaving me concerned that I could wind up stranded miles from home with no way to get back.

# Hanging on to Independence

I mean literally hanging on. One morning I was clinging to the wall in our bedroom, while my wife pulled up my pants. My knees began collapsing in slow motion. Somehow we managed to finish, but I realized I had crossed another major milestone. I was now non-weightbearing. I had been dreading this moment because I knew it meant my life was going to dramatically change once again.

For example, to put on my pants, I would need to start them over my feet, get back into bed and then roll back and forth as I pulled them further up my legs. But I was also getting too weak to roll back and forth. And sliding into bed had become so difficult that I needed the ceiling lift. I would lower the sling behind my back (with the sling already attached to the lift) fasten the chest strap and put the leg straps under my knees and hook them to the lift. Then I would use the remote control to operate the lift and pick myself up from the wheelchair. Next I would grasp a rope that crossed our ceiling and pull on it to slide over to the bed. You can see a video I made of this process on my blog site.

Now I had a new problem to solve, but my method of transferring into and out of bed might hold the solution. If I had pants that I could place flat on the wheelchair, I could lower myself onto them and fasten them around me. I could get dressed without going back to bed. But after searching online and trying several options, I had not found anything that really worked well. It was time to get out the sewing machine.

I started with one of my USA Jeans shorts and ripped out all of the stitching along the inseams and crotch so the pants would lay perfectly flat. I removed the zipper, added a little extra material to the inseams, and lined them with hook and loop. I added hook and loop where the zipper had been as well. The result was exactly what I was looking for. For once it was a solution "that had legs." I'm wearing a pair of those pants right now.

You are probably thinking (and I should have been realizing) that my condition was getting too serious for me to manage by myself. Our children had been talking with me for the past year about getting some extra help. After all, we could no longer vacuum or clean and Beth's eyesight was so poor that she could not help if I got into trouble. "Get help!" our daughters would yell, almost in unison.

Did we? Yes. Right away? Of course not. First, I had to worry about money. There actually was a lot of worrying to do. There are two ways to hire caregivers. One way costs a lot of money. The other costs a little less, and then a great deal more later.

The safest way to hire a caregiver is through a home care service. The service provides caregivers who have already been screened so you don't need to worry about their reliability, freedom from arrest records, immigration status, etc. They will also have those caregivers on their own payroll so you don't need to deal with all the extra stuff that comes along with having an employee.

The other way is to find caregivers through personal ads or by word of mouth and hire them directly. The hourly rate will almost certainly be less than what you would pay a service. However, if those caregivers work for you past a certain amount of time, they become your employees, which means you must withhold Social Security (and pay the employer share of Social Security), deduct state disability insurance, and have a workmen's compensation insurance policy. You will need to submit reports to the state and federal governments quarterly.

(What if you hire a caregiver yourself and decide to not pay any of the extras or file reports? People have done that. You frequently read about them in the news. Don't even think about it.)

When you are no longer able to work, have not saved millions of dollars and are not receiving a generous pension from a former employer, the expense of hiring caregivers can be terrifying. For that reason, we started out very cautiously. In the beginning, we only had a caregiver come in during the morning to get me out of bed, give me a shower and help Beth get dressed. That was just a couple of hours a day. Soon we realized it wasn't enough, and we hired a second caregiver to come in the evening to prepare dinner, help us get to bed, then lock up the house and leave. That amount of care is at least $40,000 annually, at least in our region, on top of living and medical expenses.

The other issue that holds some people back from getting help when they need it is psychological. They dread the idea of having a stranger coming to their house while they are in bed. They are nervous and ashamed to have a caregiver give them a shower or help them with the toilet. By now, you've probably guessed that I am one of those people.

It turned out that I was doing way too much worrying. Our first caregiver was a wonderful lady who was quite experienced with dealing with people like me. Within a couple of weeks I was wondering how I had ever managed without her. Then we hired our second caregiver, who was originally from Peru. Not only did we get the extra help we needed, we frequently got to enjoy Peruvian food for dinner. We also relied on the caregivers to drive us to appointments. So for another few months, life was not so bad.

# Words and Music

A disease like inclusion body myositis can really keep you busy. But if that's all you do or think about, it is easy to become depressed. During the years I was on the board of the San Diego Watercolor Society, I was challenged and fulfilled. Once that job was over, I could easily have hunkered down and waited for the end.

I needed something else that would keep me motivated, something that would make use of abilities I already had. I spend a lot of time on the computer and had been following several blogs about topics that interested me. One day I realized I could be a blogger, too.

When I started Life Disabled, I thought it would be a place where I could complain about bus service, talk about our life in Rancho Bernardo, and show off some of the adaptive devices I had made. It turned out to be much bigger than I had envisioned. At first, only a few people visited the blog each day.

Then I started adding videos. My audience grew and spread to the point where I was reaching people around the world. Many would leave comments and those were a source of tremendous satisfaction. Today, several thousand people visit my blog each month and tens of thousands of different individuals have visited my site at one time or another. If only one percent of those visitors found value in my blog, I feel very fulfilled indeed. In fact, I felt so good about the way things were going, I decided to express my feelings in song.

I am no singer. Ask anyone in my family and they will gladly tell you that! However I did have a bit of music in my background. I started playing piano at the age of 3 and never stopped until I was forced to by inclusion body myositis. This had given me enough music theory knowledge to be dangerous.

I started by writing a set of lyrics and worked out a melody on a miniature MIDI keyboard using my thumb, the only digit that could press a key. So now I had a song, but I needed an arrangement.

There was a new computer program called "Band in a Box." I would type in a series of chords and the program would automatically generate a backing track of instruments playing in the style and tempo that I chose. I could also type in the melody that I had composed and the program would adjust the music to fit.

The next step was to record the song, which meant (ugh!) I had to sing it. We had a spare bedroom in the far corner of the house, where I set up a microphone and would close the door and work on my song after Beth was in bed.

Finally, I put the music background and my singing into another computer program, "GarageBand," and produced the finished song. I knew the music wasn't that great so if I was going to make it public I had to add something else.

I recorded some video of me rolling my wheelchair around the neighborhood. I used the program "iMovie" to put the music and video together and then posted the result on my blog.

Finally I wrote a blog post about what I had done and linked it to the video. You can see it on YouTube, just be warned that you might want to have the sound down low. So far the video has been watched, and possibly listened to, by nearly 2,000 people. No one needs to worry about another song coming out, because my voice is now so weak singing is nearly impossible.

If you are curious, here are the lyrics to the song: (The sheet music is also available on my blog site.)

It started with a stumble,
Just a little slip, that's all
Soon each step became a struggle
And every trip became a fall
Before long I was rollin'
Down the roads I used to run
If I'd known all that was comin'
Would I just decide I'm done?
No I won't stand for that.
I'm too much man for that
I never planned for this
But life's too grand to miss
There are stories to be written
And lessons to be learned
There is beauty to be captured
And love to be returned

(Instrumental 16 bars)

Should I choose to give up early
Before this clumsy race is through?
Just lie right down and wait around
And hope my days are few?
No I won't stand for that
I'm too much man for that
I never planned for this
But life's too grand to miss

Even though I can't sing it anymore, I still believe in the lyrics.

# Who Brought the Little Girl?

The next big change to hit our life literally appeared out of thin air. It was a couple of weeks before Christmas, 2011, and we had three couples over to our house. After they left, my wife turned to me and asked, "Who brought the little girl?"

"What little girl?"

"Surely you saw her," Beth said, "She was sitting in the corner chair, but every time I looked at her she would hide behind the couch."

There had been no little girl. But no arguing would convince Beth that she had not been there. Up until that moment, I felt confident we could manage whatever came along. But this was obviously a hallucination and it signified some kind of mental issue. I hoped it would never happen again.

The hallucinations continued. They became more complex and frightening. Over time they completely took over Beth's day-to-day life. Things that used to interest her, like her favorite TV shows and creating art, no longer did. Her brain had created situations far more stimulating than any the real world could offer.

From the beginning, I thought her problems might be stemming from myotonic muscular dystrophy. It is known to cause cognitive issues. However, neither her primary care physician nor her neurologist agreed with me. They wanted her to see a psychiatrist and psychologist for the potential diagnosis of either Alzheimer's disease or schizophrenia. She underwent a three-hour-long neuropsychological evaluation that was inconclusive; she couldn't see well enough to perform many of the tasks required. Nevertheless, the neurologist suggested Alzheimer's was the cause. The psychiatrist said she could be schizophrenic and prescribed a moderate dose of antipsychotic drugs. All through this process, Beth's mental state continued to worsen.

Before long, her hallucinations and delusions caused her so much agitation, especially in the middle of the night, that neither of us was getting any sleep. For a time, she slept in the spare room, but that arrangement brought up new concerns: What would we do if one of us needed help quickly? And how could we keep her safe at night when no one else could see what she was seeing?

At this point, we realized we needed to decide whether to hire additional help – including an overnight caregiver – or move to assisted living, where there would always be help available when we needed it.

No one should have to make such a heart-wrenching decision, although hundreds of thousands of people do every year. From a strictly emotional standpoint, there was no question that we both wanted to remain in our home. But did that make sense either for our safety or financial security?

# Get Help or Get Out?

This is an important decision process and one many will face someday, so I believe it is worth going into quite a bit of detail. Perhaps the most important question is, "How long must your money last?" In our case, it was a complicated question and ultimately one that I badly overestimated. At the time, I was 71 and my wife was 64. Neither of us was in good health, but as far as we knew, my wife's illness would not dramatically shorten her lifespan. On the other hand, she was a breast cancer survivor and had several other health issues, so we couldn't count on her having a truly long life expectancy. For the purpose of financial estimating, I decided to expect her to live to be 80, and that I would probably also live to be 80. That would mean I would die 6 years before she did.

I prepared a spreadsheet showing our fixed income, which only consisted of our Social Security and my IRA. Beyond that, our assets were the house we lived in and an investment account.

There were expenses that would continue whether we lived at home or in assisted living. These included health insurance, personal liability insurance, some type of home insurance (either homeowner's or renter's), and part D Medicare insurance. There were also the out-of-pocket medical expenses, including dental care, prescription deductibles, which were quite high for my wife, and equipment expenses, most of which were not covered by Medicare. We still had the ramp-equipped minivan and we intended to keep it for independent transportation, although we needed someone to drive us. So I included gasoline, maintenance, auto insurance and license fees. I gave us each an allowance for personal items, plus estimates for gifts. We did not have any vacation expenses, but we did occasionally eat out. I also included the cost of premium cable TV, high-speed Internet access, and cell phones.

If we were to remain in the home, I would need to account for property taxes, HOA fees, landscape maintenance, a cleaning service, utilities, and an allowance for future maintenance such as plumbing repairs, roof repairs, etc.

If you make your own calculations, you may want to include the cost of travel and dining out, something we didn't need to think about.

We were getting by without taking much out of savings until we started getting home care. At the time I was making my calculations, we had two or three caregivers visiting us at different times of the day, and our total monthly cost was a little over $3,000. But that was no longer enough help. It would cost more than $8,000 a month just for the minimum help we needed. If we eventually needed help throughout the day, the total would be close to $15,000 a month. That might not seem like much for someone who is wealthy, but for us it meant our limited savings would be gone within a couple of years. Then what?

My analysis definitely pointed us toward assisted living, but assisted living is by no means inexpensive. Most facilities in Southern California average more than $100 a day for a room plus the estimated costs for care. People who need as much help as my wife and I did could expect to pay between $5,000 and $6,000 a month each. That was not financially attractive either, although when you make the decision to move to assisted living, you gain another asset: the house you are living in, if you own it.

We decided that we would try to rent our home, which, since it was paid for, would produce a better income stream. If we sold it, a safe investment such as a long-term CD would only pay about 1 percent.

However, could we find an assisted living facility that would feel comfortable, and that would accept us with our significant disabilities? I soon found that many facilities were not interested in taking me at all. The assisted living industry is built around a target market of frail elderly people, mostly in their 80s and 90s. They are not equipped to handle my physical requirements. I could not stand or walk or assist with transfers. At 6'4" and 220 pounds, it was going to take several caregivers to move me unless I could install my ceiling lifts. Most facilities had a policy that they would not accept a ceiling lift, nor would they accept a resident who was so physically disabled. Some would not even accept power wheelchairs.

Beth presented a different challenge because her hallucinations were continuing to grow worse and she was becoming a risk for getting lost. There are facilities that specialize in the kind of care she might need, but they are strictly equipped to handle people with memory or cognitive problems.

We found a couple of facilities that would accept both of us, but not in the same building. Because we would be in completely separate programs, the cost was almost as great as having 24-hour care at home. Besides, we had never been separated and didn't intend to be after spending the last 40 years together.

Some of the facilities suggested that I needed skilled

nursing since I was non-weightbearing. My wife and I helped care for my mother while she was in skilled nursing and we both knew it wasn't where we wanted to be. I liked to spend my days out running around on my wheelchair, and my wife was still interested in having a social life.

Fortunately we found Huntington Manor, a unique 27-bed assisted living facility in Poway, California, just 5 miles from our home. The owner came to our house to get to know us and make sure he understood our requirements. His facility specializes in caring for the very frail elderly, which means they are equipped to handle my physical needs, and can deal with cognitive issues. It is a cross between skilled nursing and assisted living, although it is licensed only for assisted living. There are no apartments, just single rooms. The owner suggested he could build a small wall at the end of a corridor to create a suite of two rooms for us. If we had to be in assisted living, this was our best option. I could even bring along my ceiling lifts, which I discovered later would be an enormous advantage.

What really clinched the deal was that my background in advertising was a perfect fit for the needs of the facility. They wanted a more consistent presence on the Internet so I agreed to rebuild their website, create a blog for posting resident news and facility updates, and make sure they were represented on Facebook. In addition, the owner loves to cook and enjoys sharing his suggestions for preparing food that appeals to the frail elderly. So that became another blog site for me to develop as well as a series of videos. There is a link to these sites in "Resources" at the end of this book.

Because I could help the facility, we received a very

favorable rate, which relieved my anxieties about us running out of money. However, I had not counted on my wife's condition worsening so rapidly. Soon the worries about money resurfaced.

# The Longest 5 Miles

Once we made the decision to move, and the reality of what we were doing sunk in, we endured many days and nights of second-guessing, depression and tears. When we moved to our home in Seven Oaks, we had promised ourselves it would be our final move. We really enjoyed our neighbors, our house, our yard, everything! Perhaps the worst part was packing away the things we had accumulated over decades of married life. Many of them were simply sold in a yard sale, which was especially painful. Others were distributed to our daughters. But the bottom line was that little of what we owned could come with us.

Beth could only take a few of her clothes and none of the fancy bed linens, towels or the things she had collected for entertaining over the years - there simply wasn't room. We didn't sell the house, so I promised Beth that if she got better, we would find a way to move back. That never happened.

When we compared the floor plan of the home we were leaving to those of the pair of rooms we were moving to, the necessity for even more stark choices was clear. One of the big reasons we had bought the house was for the art studio. Our proudest possession within that studio was the stack of flat files for storing watercolor materials, Beth's collage materials, and finished paintings. Now they had to go. Thankfully, my daughter agreed to store them for us.

We took most of our art supplies along, thinking that we would resume our work as artists once we settled into the facility. (I have spent the last year slowly giving away almost everything except for a set of paints and a handful of brushes. Unless there is some miraculous cure that gives me back some strength in my hands, those supplies will never be of any use to me.)

I had long ago given away my golf clubs, hunting and fishing equipment, tennis rackets, camping gear, bicycle, power tools, and everything else connected with an active life. (I don't miss the "stuff" nearly as much as I miss the life it represented.)

On May 21, 2012, my daughter drove us one at a time to our new home. The staff at the facility went out of their way to make us feel comfortable, and served us lunch at a table on the deck outside our rooms. It was a lovely setting overlooking the athletic fields of the local middle school and, farther away, the hills and mountains of Poway. If you looked closely at one hill about a mile south, you could see a patch of green grass dotted with clusters of tall trees. We didn't know it at the time, but that was going to be our final resting place, Dearborn Memorial Cemetery.

I'm sure many people wonder, "What is it like to be in assisted living?"

Ask me now and I would say that it is comfortable, a bit lonely, a good place to do some serious writing. But when we first moved in, we were excited. It was a little bit like being on vacation, except there wasn't a pool, ocean view, sightseeing excursions or minibar. That feeling lasted a few days until we realized that this was it - our penultimate stop along life's journey. The adventures were over.

For the first few weeks, we had plenty of visitors. Friends and relatives would come to see where we were. With the exception of a couple of close friends and our daughters, most people only visited once.

There was a time when we would have welcomed such a simple life. Shortly after we were together, we spent a weekend in the mountain resort of Idyllwild, about 90 miles northeast of San Diego. As we wandered the tiny village and browsed the rustic shops, we dreamed of moving there and opening a combination bookstore and art gallery. Beth would paint and I would write and we would be so happy forever after, just the two of us.

That was young love; this was old reality.

One of the big differences about life in assisted living is that much of your time is occupied with getting through the basic necessities of living. At 6:30 in the morning, pairs of caregivers would come into our rooms to begin the process of getting us ready for the day. Over in Beth's room, I would hear Adele's "Rolling in the Deep" blasting out of the boom box. It was her favorite song at the time and the caregivers liked it too. They would be singing along while they bathed her and got her dressed. It was more complicated on my side because they needed to hook me into a sling and then use my overhead lift system to raise me from the bed and lower me into a shower chair. Then they could push me into the bathroom for my shower. Afterward, they really appreciated my special wheelchair pants since they didn't need to lift me to get me dressed. Then we drove ourselves in our wheelchairs to the dining room for breakfast. Most of the other residents were not so fortunate to be able to move independently.

Breakfast was often noisy, because several residents had cognitive issues that caused them to vocalize in strange ways. One in particular would make a sound that (to me) seemed like an outboard motor trying to start up. After several weeks of hearing it, I finally realized he was repeating the Rosary over and over in an Irish brogue. It was the last of language he could still remember.

The food was excellent, and still is. But Beth had a great deal of difficulty eating because her vision was so poor and her hand-eye coordination was even worse. She also had difficulty swallowing and frequently choked, because myotonic muscular dystrophy had weakened her swallowing muscles.

After breakfast, we would be on our own. For the first couple of months, Beth was able to see well enough I could lead her on sightseeing expeditions. Within a couple of miles were a park and several shopping centers. Many days were devoted to getting to a doctor's appointment. This was complicated since we needed to use the aforementioned MTS Access.

We had lunch and dinner on the deck. A trail was directly below and horseback riders, bikers and hikers would wave to us as they passed. We waved back. It was like seeing our former selves passing by.

"Wait for us!"

# Beginning of the End

For a while I was able to convince Beth that we had left all the dangers behind when we moved. But after a few weeks, as evening approached, she would become more agitated and her hallucinations would start to take over. As the months passed, they grew more vivid and terrifying. Our daughters and I became concerned she would seriously injure herself or someone else. Finally I called her therapist, who told me to try to have her admitted into a senior behavioral unit. The therapist also made a call, and between us we were able to have her admitted within a couple of days. At the very least, we hoped that spending a few days with a multidiscipline team available to evaluate and treat her might help. However, after two weeks, the doctors said they could not determine the cause of her mental decline. They believed she should have a higher dose of antipsychotic drugs and be placed in a "memory care" facility where she would be safer.

The only way I know to describe how much this decision hurt is to reprint the blog entry I made after being given that news:

"Forty years ago, when Beth and I met, we fell so hopelessly in love we were willing to uproot both of our lives so that we could spend the rest of our years together. We were inseparable; holding hands wherever we went, even on our way to the laundromat where we would sit together and watch our clothes dry. We had two beautiful daughters, now with families of their own. I learned to share her love for art, and we began our retirement intending to spend the rest of our lives painting together. When I became disabled 15 years ago, she helped me cope. Then she became disabled a few years later, as though we needed to share that too.

For the past year or so, Beth has been leaving me. Not out the door or to the arms of another, much farther than that. Her brain is taking her slowly but certainly to a place that I cannot visit nor even comprehend. And now this terrible illness, yet to be named despite two weeks of trying by a team of UCSD doctors and psychiatrists, has progressed to the point that the unthinkable is happening. In order for her to receive the kind of care she needs and deserves, she must move to a special facility, and there is no place for me. I can visit as often as I wish, and I will. But when I return to my room, with its ceiling lifts and hospital bed and accessible fixtures, there will be no soft greeting to make this austere environment feel like home. Even worse is knowing that she will also be alone without the hope that I might rescue her from the tigers and lions, snakes and assassins and all the other evil images that come stalking as the light fades. I hope this new place and new medicine will make them go away. But even so, I know that the illness has also taken her ability to understand the reasons we are apart. Beth will only know that I am not there, and wonder why the person who once happily spent hours helping her pick curtain fabric has vanished into the murky night."

# Eleven Days of Frank Sinatra

I wish now that I'd been more questioning of the medical profession. I now believe Beth was receiving the wrong treatment and did not belong in the memory care facility. The antipsychotic medicine did not seem to be helping much. She was still hallucinating and the medicine seemed to be having an adverse effect on her breathing. The only real benefit the memory care facility offered was that it was secure so she could not roam around outside and get hurt. However, it was a "one-size-fits-all" kind of program and they treated all the residents as if they had a mental age of about 6. I may be insulting some 6-year-olds when I say this. All day long they kept the residents busy playing simple games, tossing a beach ball back and forth, and singing very old childhood songs like "Comin' Round the Mountain." This was hardly appropriate for the woman who loved Adele and had a more current music collection than my youngest daughter did.

It was a 4-mile wheelchair ride from my facility to Beth's new one, but I would try to get over there every day to spend some time with her. The best way for me to get in was through the garage elevator, and as soon as I would wheel inside, I would hear Frank Sinatra. The owner was evidently a big fan. On the eleventh day, I had a doctor appointment and could only stay for a few minutes in the morning, but I noticed Beth was much more lethargic than ever. I told the nurse to keep a close eye on her and explained my concern.

That evening I received a call from the nurse telling me they had taken Beth to the emergency room at the hospital next door. When I got there, she was unconscious and being helped to breathe by a ventilator. My oldest daughter was already there and had asked the doctor to keep Beth alive until our other daughters arrived. Beth was no longer capable of breathing on her own, and we would have to let her go unless they performed a tracheostomy and put her permanently on a ventilator. However, they warned, she probably would not regain her mental function (which was already severely compromised) and most of her organs were shutting down. Beth and I had discussed this in advance and I knew her wishes. We told them to allow her to pass away.

They removed the ventilator, gave her a strong dose of morphine, and as my daughters and I held her hands, she struggled to breathe for a couple of minutes and then her hand went completely limp. The woman who had been the love of my life for 40 years was gone.

I asked if there would be an autopsy and they said there would not, because the death was due to natural causes.

I told them her condition had been a mystery to all the doctors, and I thought an autopsy was in order.

They told me I would have to order and pay for it myself through the County Coroner. So that is what I did. I also requested a pathology report on her brain tissue. Even before I got the full report, I saw the death certificate and knew that the doctors had been wrong. The cause of death was respiratory failure due to myotonic muscular dystrophy. The neuropathology showed considerable damage to one side of her brain that had been caused by a lack of blood flow.

Myotonic dystrophy is known to cause heart

arrhythmias, which can reduce blood flow to dangerous levels and starve the brain of oxygen (hypoxia). For the past year or so, Beth had probably been having episodes of hypoxia which had been causing progressive damage to her brain, affecting her ability to reason, which, combined with her loss of vision, turned her life into a world of hallucinations.

I remembered the arguments I had with her primary care physician about the need to perform regular electrocardiograms. The doctor said it was not necessary, but eventually I was able to get my wife's neurologist to write the doctor a strong letter telling her that an EKG was part of the standard of care for myotonic dystrophy. What I did not know is that more modern practice calls for longer-term monitoring, at the least a 24-hour Holter study, because the arrhythmias come and go. It would just be dumb luck if an EKG happened to catch an arrhythmia.

# Finding Strength When You're Weak

The night Beth died, my daughter drove me back to my assisted living facility and I went to bed in my room, which suddenly seemed very small, cold and ugly. For many weeks, as grief took over, the entire world seemed to have lost any semblance of beauty. I decided to face the pain head on and created a website devoted to my wife, http://beth.shirkstudios.com. It turned out to be a wonderful solution. I produced a permanent memorial to Beth and brought myself comfort.

For the first few months, I paid little attention to my own health. In fact I told my doctors that it really didn't matter anymore since I would be happy to say goodbye. That was obviously the depression talking, and soon it was time to start dealing with my own physical status, which was growing worse. I don't know whether it was the lack of motivation or if it was just the natural progression of my inclusion body myositis, but I was rapidly growing weaker. This weakness was especially obvious in my hands and arms and in my breathing.

When you're being assessed for disability, they want to know how well you can perform various activities of daily living. Well, eating and breathing are two of the more important ones, and I was losing my ability for either one. I couldn't manage to bring a forkful of food from a plate to my mouth. Of course I was surrounded by caregivers and could become one of the people they call "feeders" – someone who is spoon-fed at each meal. There were plenty of reasons I didn't want that to happen, partly because it would cost a lot more money for me to stay there and also because I have to eat very carefully to avoid choking.

At the Muscular Dystrophy Association clinic, they recommended I try a mobile arm support. The device attached to my wheelchair and held my right forearm. Strong rubber bands neutralized the force of gravity. It helped and for a while I thought it was the perfect answer to all my problems. But before long my weakness progressed further and even with the mobile arm support I couldn't reach my mouth. I believe it was sheer desperation that led me to discover a bizarre motion I could make with my arm to sling it in a full half circle from plate, up in the air, and over to my mouth. That's the way I eat today and you can see my technique in action on my Life Disabled blog site. Just be sure not to view it around your own mealtime! While effective, the motion can have the effect of tossing food around the room. It's why I never allow anyone to sit to the left of me when dining.

The breathing issue has come as a shock, because every description of inclusion body myositis that I have seen claims that breathing is spared, unlike with some other neuromuscular illnesses. But then I found a Netherlands 12-year study of several dozen IBM patients that showed respiratory failure was much more likely to be a cause of death among IBM patients than the general population. I also found a case study of an IBM patient whose maximum inspiratory pressure (MIP) and expiratory pressure (MEP) declined over time.

I visited my pulmonologist, who ordered a respiratory function test. The results were dramatic. My ability to breathe in (MIP) was less than one-third of the low end of the normal range and in fact was below the level where ventilation is typically called for. Since this measurement is directly related to the strength of the diaphragm, it is clear that my diaphragm is much weaker than it should be. I've not had any other disease that could cause this effect. My ability to breathe out (MEP) was equally low and this explained why my speaking voice was growing weaker. MEP is related to the abdominal and thoracic muscles, which were weakening as well. The good news was that my lung function was just fine, so as long as I was breathing, my system was getting the oxygen it needed.

I returned to the MDA clinic and they suggested I get a better ventilation system than the simple BiPAP machine I had been using for sleep apnea. I eventually got one, although it took a lot of persuasion before the pulmonologists at my medical clinic would authorize it. This ventilator provides nighttime air in the volume I need rather than simply blowing air at a certain pressure. If my breathing becomes less effective during the night, the machine will make sure that I still get enough air. It also has a daytime setting which allows me to get an extra boost of ventilation anytime I am feeling tired. This is making a tremendous difference in both my alertness and my strength during the day.

There was an interesting side effect to my breathing weakness. I had been noticing that when I would try to do anything that required effort, as simple as opening a door or picking up a mug, I would hold my breath. A physical therapist told me that the diaphragm is an important muscle for maintaining posture as well as for breathing. She said my weak diaphragm was no longer able to do both things at once, so instinctively I was holding my breath whenever I did an action that required holding my body upright.

# Stay Away From Hospitals

This chapter is a reminder to myself but it is also a warning to anyone who has a disease that causes you to have difficulty walking, standing, or assisting with transfers. Through sad experience, I have learned that some medical providers are among the worst at understanding the needs of the disabled and equipping their facilities accordingly.

My pulmonologist ordered a CT scan. The radiology unit was in a state-of-the-art hospital, so I assumed they would have everything they needed to transfer me from my wheelchair onto the scanner table. That turned out to be a silly assumption. They didn't even have access to a Hoyer lift, the most basic of necessities when dealing with the disabled. The result was an awkward and dangerous process of half lifting, half dragging me out of the chair and onto the table. I would have felt sorry for the overwhelmed technicians if I weren't so busy waiting for the floor come up and get me.

That was merely an appetizer for what was to come. A few weeks later, I needed to spend one day in the hospital for an intestinal issue. I arrived in my Permobil C500 power chair. The hospital staff seemed shocked when I told them that I could not stand up and transfer; they would have to find a way to lift me.

"A Hoyer lift?" I asked.

They shook their heads. "We will get a lift team."

I expected to see a group of former NFL lineman show up. Instead, the lift team consisted of anyone who was not on break at the moment. I tried to explain that I had contractures on my left arm and left leg and that I would be no help whatsoever, not because I was unwilling, but because I couldn't. Nevertheless, they each grabbed a limb, said "One, two, three!" and lifted.

I have a fairly high tolerance for pain, and even when something really hurts I try not to make too much of it. I literally screamed out loud at the top of my lungs. But on a positive note, they didn't drop me to the floor. This process was repeated three more times until I was finally in my hospital bed.

For the next 24 hours, every time I needed to be moved, even if I simply needed a bedpan, the hospital staff would struggle and strain and in the process inflict considerable pain. They had no way of dealing with a physically disabled patient. I asked one of the nurses why the hospital was not better equipped to handle people like me. Her answer was that they had all kinds of patients, not just people like me. Of course that is true, however local grocery stores also have all kinds of people shopping, but they still manage to have wide unobstructed aisles, handicap parking out front, and automatic doors.

I wrote about my experience on my blog and it stirred up a lot of response. The theme of the comments was the same: Everyone was running into this kind of problem with medical facilities, and no one was doing anything about it. The hospital in question even asked me to meet with some of their staff about the issues I had faced. They were sympathetic, but couldn't offer any assurance that it would be fixed in the near future. I have been back twice since and nothing seems to have changed.

The problem is even worse in smaller facilities. Ironically, when I asked a leading neurologist to follow my case, he shook his head and explained that part of his office was not handicapped accessible. Every day this man was diagnosing people with progressive neuromuscular illnesses, but he did not have wheelchair access to his office! My primary care physicians over the years have never seen me out of the chair. I could have a colony of ground squirrels living on my backside and they would never know it.

About the only good thing to come from this lack of handicap access is that the local court system quickly and permanently excused me from jury duty once they learned of my physical condition.

# Being Disabled is a High-Pressure Job

As this muscle wasting disease progresses, I spend more of my time sitting and lying in one place without moving. Two of the biggest problems that result are edema, which I covered earlier, and pressure sores.

Pressure sores are ugly, painful and dangerous. They may develop quickly into a pressure ulcer that can reach all the way to bone. That will put you into the hospital for aggressive treatment to avoid sepsis, a blood infection that can destroy organs and quickly lead to death.

The best way to avoid pressure sores is to not get an illness like IBM or any other condition that restricts mobility. If you remain in one position for a long time, there will be pressure points that are bearing more than their share of your weight. In those areas, blood flow is cut off and the tissue starts to die. The most dangerous type of sore is the kind that starts deep under the skin. By the time it appears at the top layer of skin, you already have a stage III or stage IV pressure ulcer.

So far, I have been fortunate to have only one sore that progressed to stage III, but that was more than enough.

Any change of position, such as standing up from time to time, perhaps with one of the new "standing" wheelchairs, will help by returning circulation to areas that were under stress. I don't have that type of chair and I am completely incapable of changing position. In bed, I cannot even roll over to one side. So I have done several things to compensate.

During the day, I try to remember to tilt and recline my wheelchair to a horizontal position several times a day, for 15 to 30 minutes at a time. This moves the pressure points from my seat to my back. Since I spend a lot of time at the computer, I tend to get wrapped up in something I am writing or designing and several hours will pass before I remember. I probably should set a timer on my computer, but that will likely just aggravate me.

My wheelchair seat is a custom-made cushion that is created by making an impression of your bottom, which is then sent to the factory where the seat is molded. Its design is intended to make more of the downward force be absorbed in the fleshy areas while avoiding pressure where bones are closer to the skin. It helps, but it must be watched and adjusted carefully. A cushion specialist can make a pressure map when you are sitting to see whether there are any "hot spots" that need to be addressed.

At night, I found that my supposedly pressure relieving bed was still managing to put a lot of pressure on several key points. In fact my deepest pressure sore developed because of that bed. This launched another battle with Medicare and medical providers.

When I had that stage III sore, my doctor ordered home healthcare. (I had brought him a picture of it since there was no way for him to see it first hand.) A nurse came every other day to clean the wound and bandage it. She said I needed a special mattress or else the sore would just continue to get worse rather than heal. She ordered a low-air-loss alternating-pressure mattress. It consisted of a couple of dozen air bladders that would take turns filling up with air and keep any part of my body from bearing too much weight for too long. The bladders had tiny pinholes in them and allowed air to leak out. This was also important as it provided air circulation around my skin. The cost of the mattress (to Medicare) was more than $500 a month, but it certainly seemed worth it. Within a couple of months, my pressure sore was better. About a week later, the medical supply company showed up and hauled the mattress away!

"Why are you taking my mattress away?"

"Your pressure sore is better, so Medicare won't authorize you to have the mattress any longer."

"But without the mattress, my pressure sore will get worse again!"

"That's right, and then we can bring it back to you."

"This just doesn't make any sense," I thought to myself and then I went online to do research. Turned out the medical supply company representative was right. The Medicare policy really is that crazy. Fortunately, I found the very same mattress, the one Medicare was paying hundreds of dollars for each month, online for $800 total, with free shipping. So I bought it with my own money and have not regretted that decision one bit.

I am still fighting skin issues. Pressure isn't the only problem, just sitting in a wheelchair and riding around causes abrasions where skin meets clothing. One visiting nurse would bandage those abrasions and then they would get really bad! I switched home healthcare companies and the next nurse told me those abrasions should never be bandaged and should be covered with a thin layer of Desitin, just like a baby's diaper rash. I hope she's right. Otherwise I can get fussy.

# Riding, Writing and Recognition

Despite the loss of my wife and nearly all of my strength, I still keep going (at least for as long as my wheelchair batteries keep going). I give a lot of the credit for that to being lucky enough to live in a facility that can use my professional skills. My "job" is pretty simple. I ride my wheelchair around the 2-1/2 acre complex and keep an eye out for interesting photographs, videos or stories. Then I return to my room and create blog entries, email campaigns, and Facebook postings for Huntington Manor. You can see my work by starting at their website and following links to the blog. The website is http://huntington-manor.com.

When we first arrived, if I saw something interesting to photograph, I would simply hold up my iPhone and take a picture. But now I am no longer able to hold up the phone and touch the screen to take the picture. Fortunately, as the iPhone commercials used to say, "There's an App for that." Actually there are cameras for that. Surfers invented the GoPro for capturing personal point of view videos of surfing. It soon spread to skateboarders, skiers, racecar drivers, skydivers - anyone involved in activities worthy of being recorded. When I saw how small it was and that it could be worn on your forehead using a special mount, I realized I had found another adaptation. Best of all, the camera came with its own Wi-Fi network that would connect to my smart phone and then it could be controlled using the GoPro App.

The camera is fixed focus and does not have any zoom capability, but it makes up for those shortcomings with an extreme wide-angle lens and the ability to take ultrahigh resolution video and still photos with up to 12 megapixels. This means I can capture a wide area in my video and later go back with Final Cut Pro and select the area needed. Sitting at my 27-inch iMac in my room, I still marvel at the incredible editing tools I have at my fingertips. Just a few years ago a studio set up like mine would have cost $1 million or more. Mine was about $1,500, including the software.

Recently I added another App-controlled camera, the Sony QX-10. It has a 10X zoom lens, takes 18 megapixel images and weighs just 4 ounces. Between the two, I can handle most of my photo and video needs.

Being a disabled writer has also gotten easier. When I worked as a writer for a living, I could type 100 words per minute with very few errors. It seemed like the words just flowed from my mind out my fingertips and onto the page or computer screen. When I lost the ability to flex my fingers, I thought my writing career was over. I could still type, but only with the side of my thumb, and at such a slow pace that by the time I finished a sentence I forgot what I had really meant to say. That is when I gave up writing altogether and decided to take up art as a career.

No longer able to draw or paint, I am back to work as a writer and am enjoying it once again. Voice recognition technology is constantly improving. This book was written entirely with voice recognition. The program does make mistakes, but I can correct some of them through voice commands. The rest I fix the old-fashioned way, with a keyboard, except mine is an on-screen version which I can operate with the mouse.

I recently read that Dostoyevsky wrote his novels by dictating them to a transcriptionist. So did Milton and Henry James. In fact, since the typewriter wasn't invented until the mid-1800s, many authors must have dictated their work. That gives me even more encouragement to continue.

# What is Next?

When I was a teenager my father took a terrible fall. He was inspecting the attic of our newly built home, stepped in the wrong place and fell all the way through to a flight of stairs in the garage. His leg was fractured in many places and after six months had not healed properly.

His doctor did a bone graft, which meant he had to return to the hospital for several weeks. One day, the hospital staff was transferring him back to his bed and dropped him, fracturing his pelvis where the graft had been taken. This meant he would spend many more weeks in the hospital. It also meant he was likely to lose his job.

Shortly after the fall, his best friend came to visit and asked my father how he was.

"If I had a gun, I would probably shoot myself," he said, "but then again, I'm curious to see what's going to happen next."

I share my father's sense of curiosity. So I will try to stick around to see what's going to come next, especially now that the human genome has been catalogued offering so many new possibilities for disease treatments.

When I was diagnosed with inclusion body myositis in 1996, my doctor and I agreed that it was pointless to try any of the drugs available at that time as trials had shown them to be ineffective, and experiences had shown that their side effects could be very serious. Once in a while new ideas would be brought forth, but I always evaluated them from two criteria: Did their mode of action seem to make sense for this particular disease, based on what we knew about its behavior? Had any studies been done that produced empirical data supporting their claims?

There were numerous anecdotal testimonials, but I discounted those since IBM is such a slow-moving disease and since our physical performance can vary so much over time due to psychological influences and general health. In other words, placebo effects could easily fool a person into thinking a regimen was working.

As of the beginning of 2014 there are three potential therapies that may hold promise. In Australia, researchers are using a fatty acid compound that can be taken orally. It is meant to increase the amount of energy available to muscle cells and slow or stop the deterioration of muscle cells.

In an Ohio clinical study, patients' muscles were injected with a follistatin transgene. This study was quite limited, but another study with mice had promising results.

The biggest news was when a new drug from Novartis (BYM338) was given breakthrough status by FDA. From what I have read, the mode of action seems to make sense. They believe they have identified an enzyme that restricts the development of new muscle cells, and that it is an overabundance of that enzyme that causes IBM patients to lose strength. BYM338 blocks the action of the enzyme, allowing muscle cells to reproduce unchecked. The drug has been through two stages of clinical trials including one that showed significant benefits when compared to a placebo. Now they are launching phase 3, which will be a much larger trial. Since the drug has received breakthrough status, a smaller proportion of trial participants will be receiving placebos, so if you are in the trial, there is a better chance you would be receiving the real thing.

My doctor at the MDA clinic called the researchers on my behalf to see if I could get into the trial. Due to my advanced stage of disease, I am non-ambulatory, and that is an exclusion from the trial. They use the 6-minute walk test as a method of determining drug effectiveness, a standard test used in many different types of illnesses. On the other hand, one of the reasons they received breakthrough designation is that this illness is life-threatening in its later stages. It may be a little unfair that they do not include a trial that focuses on those of us who are at those late stages and may not have time to wait for general availability of the drug. I have already been waiting 18 years; I'll try to hold out a little longer.

# Rewriting Life's Script IBM Style

I believe that most of us carry a script in our minds. It will be different for everyone, depending on where we were born, what our parents were like, what our teachers thought of us, and so on. The point is, this script tells us where we think we are going to be at each stage of our life. I was born in a small town in Indiana; my parents struggled through the Depression and managed to have a comfortable middle-class existence. I was fortunate enough to go to college, get a good job when I came out, and begin living a typical middle-class life.

My script had modest expectations. I would get married, work until I was retirement age, own a nice home, raise brilliant and successful children, and retire near a lake and a golf course. Oh, and I would write the Great American Novel.

The script was working out fairly well, the leading characters were doing their parts, and then I got inclusion body myositis.

Throw that script in the bonfire! When I was first diagnosed, I soon realized that my script needed a serious rewrite. Of course that was only the beginning. That script has been rewritten so many times, I've completely run out of erasers, and my delete key is worn to the nub. But I think this is a good thing.

When we don't rewrite our life script despite bad things happening, we are setting ourselves up for a life of depression and worry. Sometimes terrible things happen almost instantly, such as an accident or the sudden death of a spouse. Other times, the change is gradual. A diagnosis of a slowly progressive disease such as inclusion body myositis or myotonic dystrophy means your life is going to change, but not right away. The changes may be imperceptible at first, almost like life itself.

In every case, life changes, and it means our script needs to be modified as well. There may be a few people who manage to make it all the way through life without needing any rewrites. I guess that could also be a good thing, but I'm not sure. There's something to be said about being challenged and being forced to find ways to adapt to a life you didn't plan.

My wish for you is that no matter how many times you must rewrite your life's script, you are satisfied with the ending.

# A Timeline of Disability

From the time my symptoms first appeared until today, the difference in my strength and abilities is astonishing. When I look at pictures of myself taken in the late 1980s and early 1990s, it is like I am looking at a totally different person. When my caregiver comes to get me up in the morning, he or she has to first drag me over to the center of the bed because my left side is so weak I will be slumped completely over against the guardrail. I can't budge from that position on my own. Compare that to the prior me who was running his own business and running half marathons (and that one fateful full marathon).

I can testify that the description of inclusion body myositis in the medical literature is quite accurate. They say it is slowly but relentlessly progressive. It is very difficult to tell from one week or even one month to the next that anything is changed. Sort of like the hour hand on a clock, which never seems to move while you are looking at it.

To help the newly diagnosed have an idea of what to expect, I have compiled the following summary of the changes I experienced and the kinds of adaptation they inspired, year-by-year.

### 1985-1995 (Pre-Diagnosis)

Stumbling while jogging
Golf club flying out of hands
Difficulty rising with backpack
Jogging speed declining

## 1996

Diagnosed at UCSD Medical Center

## 1997

Started using walking sticks to help avoid falls

## 1998

Purchased scooter for distances more than 100 yards,
Purchased van with lift in rear for scooter

## 1999

Fitted for full leg braces (KAFO) and forearm crutches
Purchased Jazzy wheelchair with elevating seat
Had condo modified with ramps at curb, entrances,
sunken living room
Replaced Roman tub with roll-in shower, added roll-up
counter in kitchen
Bought fiberglass portable ramp

## 2000

Purchased raised toilet seat
Purchased hand controls for van
Retired on disability
Gave up piano, golf, tennis, took up watercolor

## 2001

Coordinator for paint-out group of San Diego Watercolor
Society

## 2002

Membership Director of San Diego Watercolor Society

## 2004

International Exhibition Director of San Diego
Watercolor Society
Purchased van with ramp and transfer seat
Took last trip with Beth

## 2005

Purchased Pride lift chair
Began making hooks and dressing sticks
Purchased grabbers (6)
Beth erroneously diagnosed with ALS
Beth correctly diagnosed with myotonic muscular
dystrophy
Acquired Permobil C500 (Medicare) for Mike
Purchased Jazzy 1103 wheelchair for Beth

## 2006

Purchased BioBidet
President San Diego Watercolor Society
Purchased single-story home
Added 200 feet of outside sidewalks for wheelchair
access
Built ADA bathroom
Acquired hospital bed

## 2007

Began using shelf liners to lift legs
Purchased wheelchair pants from USA Jeans
Past President/Technology Director of San Diego
Watercolor Society

## 2008

Purchased ceiling lifts for bedroom and bathroom just in case

## 2009

Purchased rechargeable wine opener (and used it a lot!)

## 2010

Purchased iPad for drawing
Purchased automatic can opener, jar opener
Purchased computerized sewing machine (no foot pedal)
Made belly bag, art apron, cooking apron, robe, work table, sliding pad

## 2011

Started using overhead lifts
Sewed pants that fastened around me after being lowered onto them
Hired part time caregiver for showers
Lost ability to drive, began relying on the bus
Hired second caregiver
Beth began hallucinating

## 2012

Moved to assisted living and put home up for rent
Beth died of respiratory failure due to myotonic muscular dystrophy
Lost most strength in arms, began using mobile arm support
Diagnosed with chronic respiratory failure

## 2013

Purchased remote controlled cameras
Purchased low air loss/alternating pressure mattress
Began writing a book

## 2014

Published "Rolling Back"

# Resources

You won't find much in the way of printed material in my resource list. I can no longer turn the pages of a magazine, let alone hold a book in my hands. So I rely heavily on my tablet readers and my computer. The following are some of the websites and organizations that I found most helpful.

Access Medical
http://www.accessmedicalrehab.com
Author's recommendation for a rehab wheelchair provider

Ability Center
http://abilitycenter.com
Mobility dealer that sold us our vans

Beth Shirk
http://beth.shirkstudios.com
Memorial for the author's late wife

Bill Tillier IBM Site
http://www.ibmmyositis.com
A site loaded with medical information

BraunAbility Voice
http://www.braunability.com/abilityvoice
News from the company that built our Braun Entervan

CircAid
http://www.circaid.com
A San Diego Company specializing in unique
compression garments

Huntington Manor Assisted Living
http://huntington-manor.com
Mike Shirk's home

Life Disabled
http://lifedisabled.com
My blog contains hundreds of photographs and videos

Muscular Dystrophy Association
http://www.mdausa.org
Research funding and patient support for more than 40
disabling illnesses

Myo Musings
http://www.myomusings.com
Personal account about living with Inclusion Body
Myositis

Myositis Support Group
http://www.myositissupportgroup.org
An informative website with a forum

Myotonic Dystrophy Foundation Community Forum
http://www.community.myotonic.org
Forum for those diagnosed with Myotonic Dystrophy and
their caregivers.

National Institutes of Health
http://www.nih.gov
Start here to research any rare illness and find clinical trials

Pacific Mobility
http://www.pacificmobility.com
The company that helped me with my ceiling lifts

San Diego Watercolor Society
http://sdws.org
Internationally recognized art organization

Shirk Studios
http://shirkstudios.com
Art created by Mike and Beth Shirk

The Myositis Association
http://myositis.org
Provides research funding for myositis muscle diseases.

USA Jeans
http://www.wheelchairjeans.com
Pants designed for sitting (as in a wheelchair)

Wheelchair Dancers
http://www.wheelchairdancers.org
A site to lift your spirits and get you moving

## How to Connect with Mike Shirk

I look forward to hearing from you.

If you enjoyed my book or found it useful, please leave a review on the seller's website.

You can visit my blog, http://lifedisabled.com and leave a comment or question.

Or visit my Life Disabled Facebook page.

Or email me at: mike@lifedisabled.com.

Or hang around the streets of Poway, CA and catch me as I roll by!

Made in the USA
Charleston, SC
07 June 2014